The *L*ove Touch

Frank L. Clark, M.D.

iUniverse, Inc.
Bloomington

The Love Touch

iUniverse books may be ordered through booksellers or by contacting:

iUniverse
1663 Liberty Drive
Bloomington, IN 47403
www.iuniverse.com
1-800-Authors (1-800-288-4677)

ISBN: 978-1-4620-7237-8 (sc)
ISBN: 978-1-4620-7238-5 (ebk)

Printed in the United States of America

iUniverse rev. date: 12/05/2011

The Love Touch will teach you how to touch the whole body; ultimately, allowing the largest organ of the human body [the skin] to come alive with positive health changes.

In Acknowledgment

Research has always been interesting to me; however, each project brings exciting new understandings, and insights. That comes from books, the internet, family, and friends. Without them, these consuming and daunting projects could not come to its reality.

I am thankful for friends, who trusted my thoughts about touch and allowed me time to demonstrate the art of touch that was needed. In touching them, I noticed changes, innovative levels of knowledge and understanding. Ultimately learning that touch has a long standing health-service history. It is important to teach The Love Touch and tell others the good news.

The 5000-year history of healing touch gives us great insight to share touch with modern medicine. We are all Humans: and we are all the same in our needs for touch, however we are different in our customs, in our character, and in our taste.

Acknowledgment

Foreword

The 21st century America have been great stresses; 50 to 60 times worse than just two years ago. Therefore, our physical needs for daily touch are great! It so doesn't it seem wise to have a powerful non-pharmaceutical therapy to address modern-day stress. Before it becomes a series illness?

We have tried it all; modern medicines, drugs, herbs, comfortable chairs, expensive mattress, latest houses, new-fangled phones, latest computers and e—mails, extra cars, new-found friends, different husbands and another wives. Things can never take the place of physical touch! What comes with The Love Touch is trust and understanding. What a different day this would be if you and I would take the touch into our busy stressful lives. Let's look towards the simple and gain great insights to what would give us *peace*.

CONTENTS

THE
LOVE TOUCH

Introduction

As a medical doctor, I have treated thousands of sick and/or diseased patients, whom are looking to their physician for clear answers? Patients ask, "Will. I get better," "Will. I make it through this illness and become well again?" Patients eventually take on the subjective ownership of a given disease, because of the attitude of their physicians and their fear. I believe that a good physician will touch their patient in times of fear, giving warmth, understanding and hope in addition to diagnosis and prognosis.

Today Life-style physicians teach lifestyle change that includes the whole-body, mind and soul, while still promoting water, fiber-rich-foods, exercise and daily touch!

In the 80s physicians' magazines had many articles that dealt with the importance of touching patients. Hundreds of times I was tooled: "You act like you care about us, Dr. Clark." I come from a touching, hugging family. Most importantly touch has always been part of my physician's mannerisms.

An East Indian Lady told an American Physician that she could not trust the doctors if he could not touch her. Touch from a person in power is very important to encourage trust. We will learn that trust takes away fears and can be simple attain with The Love Touch.

The Love Touch Beginning!

One must understand how the love touch came to be! It did not just appear, but came by the ways of learned experiences, while keep my heart intone to the needs of others. Accordingly, this adventure gives bases for the love touch, while at the same time allowing us to embrace touch in a very special moment.

The few minuets spent here will only give you merit to study touch and learn why it is so important to our everyday lives. I have learned for this research that I need touch daily, too!

Beginning 101:

I was born in the winter. Mother was a musical lady, who played the piano daily for school children. She played for evening's worship at home, church on Sabbath and Sundays, coral practice on Friday night, and many other public singing service events. Moreover, she was an accomplished musician, who played large pipe organs; The Institute of Detroit Art Museum, St. John's, and many others sizable churches and institutions in the Detroit area.

Mother, whom I ultimately know from the inside made my life delightful. This allowed me to know first-hand the sounds of her musical style. So, my first love touch is here mother and music. How do I know that, because when I sing a song that I have heard for many years it comes to my brain and when I think about sing the song and the pitch, words, and melody are there? I sing a delightful, fun-loving song, and the methods with her diction come through. Music is one of the best activities on the Earth; yes, it is alive and real!

Mother returned to work when I was old enough to stay overnight with my grand-parents. They lived five miles from my parent's home. There, my mother's parents care for my needs. I learned the love touch while sitting on my grandfather knees and sitting next to him at the meal's time. I sit on his lap, while he drives his truck to the end of the drive way, to go to work. Grandma would get me out of the truck. We would walk back to the house. She would feed me breakfast, and then showed me how shining her wood tables' legs.

Grandparents/my parent taught me to appreciate a good-healthy life-style. This includes fresh garden vegetables, colorful fruits, lots of water and daily walks to the woods.

Often Mother would come home and find me playing on napping Dad's lap. Dad always touched us boys (my brothers) by tucking us in bed and hugging us when we came home or was leaving. Runny nose, sore throat, and puny feeling would make me sick. Dad would place a cool wash cloth around my nick in a hand toll to secure it. Dad rubbed my chest and the bottoms of my feet with Vicks vapor rub. Then I put on clean socks and fresh wasted t-shirt . . . all to make me feel better. I was love touched! In the morning, I felt refreshed and healthy.

On special-occasion—Thanksgiving and Christmas, I cut vegetable for meals! Mother and I listen to classical music while preparing healthy foods that our families like to eat. I enjoy cooking, because food is satisfying and prevents over eating. Properly seasoned natural foods affect our taste buds differently than fat, sugary, calories in processed foods.

On these special-occasions family members would come from Cleveland, Ohio; Washington DC, Nebraska, Hawaii, and other parts of the country. There were lots of hugs and kisses on coming in and leaving. We were eaten at a large table, and the social times and foods were the best, because it came from our gardens, and we made home-cooked meals. I loved all of it. Best of all was great communications that strengthen are trust and love for each other.

Mother taught me to turn music pages, while she practiced or performed. I was small, but I enjoyed the grandiose pipe organ sounds; especially when mother played classical music with full peddles it made the building swell with great joy!

Activities of lives help shape my thoughts about the love touch. Gardening gave me different insight of caring touch from the other chores; like making my bed, washing dishes, cleaning off the table. Logical thinking comes from gardening; it's natural and math is used; meaning I learned to tile the earth with grace. The rolls had to be straight; the rolls had to be even, and they needed planting, watering, holding and weeding. Carrots were the hardest, because when they came up, they looked the same weeds. While learning to identify weed and carrots, I took a hand filled with weeds and carrots and tossed them. I thought about it and changed my thoughts about just doing it that way. So, I was waiting a day, and then weeded, and it worked well! Now, I loved to weed carrots, because I can visualize good results; beautiful taste vegetables. Since then I always looked forward to summer garden; corn on the cob, fresh snapping green bean, yellow squish, okra, and mashed potatoes; sliced beef steak tomatoes, rudder beggars, onions, and tomatoes.

Often, I walked the dirt roads to the Creek, not very far from home. There, I watched the sand dollar crayfish working in the mud on the banks of the Creek; water spiders danced across the water, without music, on their anatomical skates. I spent enjoyable times their; in the summer swimming and winter ice skating. Spearing carp was big in the farming country, in the early spring; and the carp speared were weights 8 to 12 pounds. Painted turtles and snapper were a plenty, too!

Bicycle riding down a dirt road was fun, and I saw flowers. Many farm animals, plenty of beautiful country farm lands. Other times I would visit farm areas and see new crops, young farm animals; then I would walk through the woods and along the rail road tracks. The dirt roads would lead to paved roads that wandered their way to Carleton, Michigan. There, I would play baseball, and visit neighbor friends going to and from the town. Drinking frosted root beer from a frozen mug was one of the high points of my day. Then I would go into Booths a 5 & 10 cent store. There were many kinds of toys for children their; games, puzzles and many different kinds of books; I liked day dreaming there. The old wooden floors in Booths would creak when I walked on them, and the ceiling had tin pattern's squares. One of the neighbors close to town had a Model-t Ford with running boards. We sit on the running boards for a while and talked. The Bajor's were sweet corn farmers and lived on the last corner on the way home. There I would visit and pick corn while riding in the wagon. Large wagons would be unloaded into Semi truck; that would take the corn to market. These were fun days, and I enjoy it.

Grandpa Copening asked one summer my three brothers, and I helped removing nails from old boards; that he would use to build rental homes. These were fun and exciting days. I got to use crowbars, hammers, and nail removal tools. It was early spring, and mornings were chilly; Grandpa had a bucket-fire to keep us warm. These work days started at 7 am. And Grandma Copening would come out about 10 am and ask if we were hungry? I was born with an empty stomach! I enjoyed her cooking, for it was healthy and delouses. By noon Grandma Copening, would call us in order to eat taste foods and drink her distinct brown sugar lemonade. I like her lemonade, because it was special.

Dad was a home builder, and he allowed me to work with him and my uncle Jim; who were a Mason and pumper? They taught me safety rules, while working with power tools. Safety worked together with being ready to handle materials, supplies, and /or tools in work area. So, that work always continued at a smooth pace; better known as anticipate the next move, while working on the jobs. Late,

I learned that this same effort work in the operating room; know as team work. Dad and Uncle Jim build many housed. I learned how to work with wood, cement, blocks, sender block, bricks, tubing, plastics, dry wall, insulation, poring side walk and basements, and even large recreation paved area for schools. I enjoyed working with Dad and Uncle Jim; this allowed me to work with Grandpa Copening at times, when he needed help to building a home.

Dad had piles of sawdust near the table-saw, while cutting woods' pieces for tomorrow's work. So I learned that I could light them, and the fire would smother. Then I would take a stick of wood and through the saw dust into the night air. The burning saw dust mixed with the night air would crackle, pop and sprinkle like home-made fireworks. Additionally, I took cat tails and soaked them in gasoline over night and light them at night the next day. They were the great home-made flayer.

With Dad's scrape wood I make sail-boats and floated them in the ditch when it rained. Designing small sail boats was enjoyable.

I was allergic to poison ivy and got it often in the spring. I even got it late winter when I make angels in the ditch one year. When I went to little legion baseball, my friend did not know me, because my face would be swelling. I out grow this allergy as I got older.

I enjoyed doing roof's jobs, because it was elevated and early in the spring morning Bob White would be singing enjoyable bird calls. The Morning dew would be on the wood and roof products; however, this did not stop me from working, because I really enjoy the mornings. One time while roofing Dad asks me to get a 2 by 4. So being proud of myself, I selected a 2 by 4. I climbed the ladder and give it to my dad, who stated," Frankie. I need a straight one." I ask, my dad, "how do you know," and" he stated just a minute, and I will come down and show you. This time he came down off the roof and showed me how to look down the length of the board. Which meant Dad allow me to view the shape down the length of the board to determine if it is either curved or looked straight. Now I could find a right board and accomplish what was needed. Dad was always kind. Dad, taught good instruction around the home, at work and every day of my life, while grow up. Dad taught me patience and kindness, too!

I spent many days and nights on Uncle Jimmy a Dairy Farm. An experience there was very different feeling, while milking the cows. The barn areas were constructed to make the cow faced each other when they came in opposite sides of the barn. This allowed us to walk in front of the cows to place feed; this keep cows busy eating, while they were being ready to be milked. This took place twice a day, morning and evening . . . everyday. First time I recall (4 years old) walking down the walk way in the winter, I could see their breath and the slime of the cows' tongue in their nose. A lot of raw energy came up on me, and it was really different. Soon, I felt that walking in front of the cow was safe. Sometimes I would feed them. As I got older I could walk behind the cow and learn safely, because they have hard broken bone kicks and hurtful tail swishes or back-u or side movements. After learning safety, I learned to wash utters so that tips would be cleaned ready for the milking machine cups.

As I got older I would go to the fields at milking times [6 am and 4 pm] with my cousins, Uncle Jimmy and the sheep dog, Buckey. Buckey was black with white spots. He was trained to bring in the cows. My Uncle gives the command, "sick emu Buckey," and Buckey would move quickly to snap at the hocks of the cows; they would come a running! Buckey was fast and that make the cow move towards the barn in top speeds.

Calf births were exciting, because I always enjoy science and nature; visualize it first hand was worthwhile. When calves are old enough to be taught to feed, I would put my finder in their mouth, and the calf would suck my finder. Thus, the calf learned to suck! What a different and net experience. It did not take very long for them to learn how to feed. I sure liked feeling the young calf's coat. It was soft and delightful the touch. Love my experiences on the farm.

Why do I tell you about my younger life? It's because the adventure into life, the farm, teaches real emotions and feeling that I could not have received from regular life. We became what we have experienced. I am grateful for caring relatives, who have taught me to care about others and the service of other. These experiences give me purpose as well as strengths to live by and take the best of the experiences while moving on!

Silage comes from chipped up field corn. It is wet with natural sugars. It is the common feed used alone with hay in the winter time. I like climbing up the ladder on the inside of the barn, where the silo was attached. It was an adventure to climb to the top, where the level of silage was at its peak. Silage has its own sweet smell and walking on it is like a walk on a bog; a setting for an adventure there.

When I got old enough to drive the tractors, I could fuel them, check the oil and attach wagons. I learned to plugs and dice, too. The gas tank was the old upright clear tank, and it had to be pumped before gas came. I loved driving in the fields, and while billing hay. I recall being 12 years old and thronging 100 lbs bile. Baling Hay bales made me money to spend at the Monroe County Fair in August each year. Baling Hay also made me strong and healthy.

Butch, my cousin owned a white horse that he allowed me ride when I visited him. Sometime, we would ride with his neighbors, who own a black horse that was fast. We played cowboys and Indian often. One time I was on the back of my cousin horse, and I went to shoot the neighbor. The horse took off, and I rolled off the horse down into the large ditch. I did not get hurt. What an adventure it was that day!

Making money on the farm was great! I take a large knife and cut the corn out of the soy bean. This occurs when they would plant soy beans after raising a field of corn. It was hard and would take all day to clean one 10 acre of soy bean. I liked cut out the corn with a knife it was adventitious, and it makes me money for the county fair.

Aunt Alpha would cook the buckwheat pancake on the old wooden stove at the farm. They were large and taste, and they used real butter and maple syrup . . . it was delicious! One time Buckey caught a cold and was sick, so my other Uncle Walter, who lived on the farm heated the wood stove hot. He instructed us children to stay away from it. Then he wrapped Buckey in a burlap bag and placed him behind the inflamed wood stove. About 1 hour later they remove Buckey and him as ringing wet and very weak, but much improved.

I loved the farm, because it was outdoors and full of nature. I learned that working the farm gives satisfaction. What fun and delightful emotions come from doing something good for the farm.

Saturday nights on the farm were special. We watch TV; eat popcorn from a large white porcelain bowl with a glass of pop. Before bed, I would have to bath and in the bathroom, they had been warming light. Warming lights are the red lights used in the chicken coop to keep the young chicks warm. Warming light had a timer on it, and I would turn it on and the warmth of the lights would fill the room, while I dried off. I liked that, because you never were cold after a bath: but it refreshed.

Grandma Copening's baths were much different, because she would sub me with castle soap. It was ruff soap, but it would shine up my knees and remove the dirt from my fifty skins. Now after this bath was a thin cup experience. Grandma would tell me to rinse with icy water to help my immune system be strong and stay away from common colds and diseases. This is the opposite of the farm, but feels good in a very different way. I appreciated the variety of opposites taught me, for it gives me choices that give me new experience in my life to make it better.

One summer while taking driver's education, the couch, who was the driver's instructor, asked me paint the bleacher at Airport High School while making money. So after driver training classes and driving, I painted the bleacher red. Now this activity gave me gas money!

Now, I had hot rods, with a fast engine that drank plenty of gas. So I worked after school and on a weekend at a gas station in Monroe, Michigan. Gas was cheeped (12 cents/gal.). I loved working there, because there were a lot of repeat customs, who I know and talk to, while pumping their gas. At the station, I learned from Tony and older man how to toast quarter against the wall. I would win sometime, however, learned that it was a waste of time. Additionally, I learned that drinking doesn't pay, because Tony would get drunk and lost his Volkswagen bug; every Friday night after we closed the station. I worked with other young men, who own Honda's Motor Bike. Often, I would ride the Honda to town for our lunches. Driving the Honda's 125 was fun, because it was small, fast, and I could feel the moving air over my body when I traveled to town.

On one different day, Jim a young working station found a cat hiding in the bushes. He wanted to know if cats have nine lives, so he felled up a trash can with water and held the cat there until it could not breathe. Then he pulled it out. The cat lived. Then he put gas on the cat, and the cat ran away. Why do young boys have to do unnecessary things to find out—what might happen?

In the fall of one year, I saw pheasants in the front yard of our county home. So, I got Dad's 16 gauge shot gun and shot the pheasant. I did not enjoy this experience! I told myself that I will on no account kill another animal.

Mason Uncle Jim had chicken that they had to rise to kill and eat them. They were our neighbor, so I saw their often. This day he killed the chicken with an ax. The chicken would run around with no head. Funny, but I did not like this. I like eating chickens, but not the killing part.

During high school, I learned to drink cheap dollar wine and smoked rum soaked cigars. Coca mama wine was treated with kola. We would drink beer, when we could get someone to buy it for us. When 2 am came, I was to be at home, because after 2, it was too late . . . according to Dad. I would be hungry, so I would get left-overs out of the refrigerator and would be eating when Dad would come in the kitchen and ask me," how was I doing?" and then sit and talk with me. Dad knew that I had been drinking and never brought it up. Dad taught me the art of communication. He could talk to anyone and any animals. Bad dogs were his friend. He could make cats climb ladder and jump over his lead-out arm. I learn that caring. Patience's and understandings are important in communications.

Some of our adventure took us to T-town [Toledo], where we drink 3/2 beer at 18 years of age. This was weak beer at clubs, and old fire stations turned into a bar (party places). With these friends and we traveled by car to Florida for spring break. First time in Florida I got sun burn on my face, learning that wearing sun screen is important. Love the fresh Orange Juice there.

Oh, I learned to smoke Camel's cigarettes for four years. I helped a friend from Canada push his car out of snow. I became short of breath; I saw stars! So, I quit smoking and never when back to that bad habit.

During my teenage years, I would ride on Woodard Ave. on Saturday night with friends, whom owned hot cars. This was a lot of fun, because I would see all types' hot-rod classics. I enjoyed bike shows and auto shows, where school friends had exhibits. I like cars and enjoy taking photos and visiting with the owners, while learning about their rides.

Henry Ford Community College, Dearborn, was my first college, where I meet Detroit and Canadians. This was a distinguishable and new-found experience and I like it, because people are so distinct I learn to tolerate, and have understanding; communications at in a peaceful way!

Then I went to Eastern Michigan University, where I receive a BS in Biology/Chemistry. This was the time for Rock Roll, Coral Music and the newness of water beds. I traveled to Europe with Eastern Michigan University Choir. We sang in Pairs, and Austria. I flow to Northern East Germany, where I visited an exchange student and her family. Heidi had been an exchange student in Monroe the summer before. This was a great adventured to older Germany, eat the foods, saw the county side and experience life in an area that was divided. They took me to the dividing line and told me that they had relatives on the other side. They also took me to a restaurant, where I had traditional German food. German apple pie is much different than American's apple pie. German's apple cake is much larger and looks more like a cake, but really tastes.

EMU Choir flow from Detroit two Pairs, France, there we visited for five days. We traveled by train through the Alps Mountains to Austria; it was beautiful and a delight to see. We sang as the train moved up the Alp's it as heartwarming to see and feel. It was hard to believe that war took place here.

After graduation, I taught histology at Easter Michigan University. I worked in Industrial Clinics as a tech, doing X-rays, suturing wounds, and giving minor shots. I enjoyed clinical experienced, because it gives more insights to the future. Teaching Histology taught me about the smallest structure of human tissue.

Pontiac Osteopathic Hospital respiratory department taught me therapy, and further clinical insights. I assisted surgery residents from Wayne State Surgery Department at the Frank Fitzsimons dog medical research lab in Pontiac. We operated on toxic dog's lungs for transplants to another dog. Testing survival results in dogs was to see if children who ingest gas and/or paint products could ultimately survive.

Wayne State University Medical School was exciting, because it was where I had always wanted to be. I wanted to learn how to heal the ill patient. I worked full-time at nights and weekends at Industrial Clinics. I had time to study when it was not busy. I was also treasure of medical note service, that medical student paid for and received typed note twice a week in the first two years.

After freshman medial school year, I worked in a Pathology workshop at Mount Carmel Hospital. There, I learned to fix and freeze tissue as well as read prepared tissue slides. This was a great medical path-experience, and I enjoy it. While taking the summer workshop at Mount Carmel, I met a Philippines resident, who taught me to cut tissue for pay at a Northville lab. So I dictated and cut tissue several days a week when the resident could not make it. Other times I would be a denier on autopsies. Denier is one who cut biopsy tissues for pathological study. While I learned making money sure help with the expenses of Medical Education.

Clinic and pathology were in the second years. I was president of the classes, treasure of Scribed Notes Service, tech at Industrial Clinics and married. You might believe that this is a lot, however, working, while in studies was my make-up. I had to do, what was necessary to keep a float in this expensive world? My work was always related to the Para medical worlds, which help in practicing and understanding medicine.

Hospital's rotations were the third year. I worked Industrial Clinics on a weekend. I was elected an Escalapian, which mean I represented my class to the Medical School Board once a month. Most important activity was put together the Mason Lodge party at the end of each year. This was a colossal fun time, because these classes put on a mocked play about medical clinic actions or problems. My freshman year the second-years class grows excitement and extravagant enacted with snap, crake and papal . . . experience; one walk across the stage acting likes a woman speculum with the movement of his arms; another was rod bacteria lying on the hospital bed and enacted sick from that bacteria; the third student enacted snapping of bone as an orthopedic doctor. This was always one of the high nights at School, because you communicated with staff from the DMC and surrounding area.

The senior year was short. I had completed my entire requirement for the medical degree by January. As a result, I started an internship in February and attended medical graduation in June of the same year. Immediately, I was starting the internship in February, because Wayne State Medical School has good instructors and teaches heavy in the clinic setting experiences.

February, I started working at Little Travis Hospital in Petoskey, Michigan as an Emergency Physician. Several times a year, I traveled North of Petoskey to work at Clinics owned by our hospital group. Anna second child was born here. She liked going to the bank often to get a sucker. Petoskey and its surrounding area are second and third homes to the very wealthy. Emergency medicine treated the high class; however, when you make a diagnosis family member would be on the phone to Mayo and other big centers. They talked to family/special doctors about the situation [diagnosis]. Then there were the local people and neighbors, whom were much easier to deal with? Northern Michigan's is God's country; it is so beautiful and rewarding to visit and/or live.

Petoskey was a tremendous place to live, because of the snow sports. There is a great nature walk in the hills where I would see wild birds and view the Grand Travis Bay, which was such a wonderful site. Casey and Anna ice skated and other snow games,. in our back yard!

Benton Harbor/St. Joseph Emergency Room was my new ER experience. It was a much different ER more middle class and very poor people. I started riding horses weekly. I liked riding at night it helped me relax after a 12 hours working a day. I was learning how to fly fix wing planes then joined a flying club. I joined the Berrien County Sheriffs Poses. The BCS Poses rode horses in parades and parked the cars the week of the Berrien County Youth Fair.

MEC+1 a walk-in clinic came two years after working the Benton Harbor/St Joseph ER, It was a sole practice. It started slow with 15 patients per day, within three months it was 50 and within nine months 100 patients per day. I was busy; however, I had several good workers. Works, who could take X-rays, give shots, put on wraps, dispense medications, give instruction and do therapy and allergy shots. The patient said that I acted like I cared! There were always 8-10 patients in the line up in front of the clinic every day at 8 am, and I worked until 8 pm. I was tired when I got home, except my two girls wanted a horsey back on me; until I was ringing wet. We laughed and play together every night. We would get in the hot tube/swim in the pool. Then I would read to them at bed time story and pray with them. T I would turn off the lights and just float in the swimming pool; great for relaxing the muscle. These were grand times!

Twelve years, I worked very hard and had many good times and events: "Inspection STD"; this was about the Aide Epidemic and VD problems "Earease" invented a non-medical device and was patented.

Michigan State Police investigated me for writing medicine outside the normal course of medical, by a complaint. Unknown by the people who started the investigation that I had o 3 percent of 25,000 patients received pain medicines. I want to say that jealously run rampant in medicine.

ATF Auto weapons were brought unknowing to me and writing medicine outside the normal course of medicine by the Michigan State Police.

FCI Milan/ Federal Correction institutions are where I was incarcerated. This was very different, because now I listen to jail and prison talk and uneducated attitudes. I learn to stay by myself, playing lots of tennis, played electric bass or organ in several bands once a week. I taught public speaking in the day school. I learned to paint art with acrylic's paints in the day school. Once a day I ran over one ½ hours. I was known as the queasy doctor, because I ran so much and stay to myself. Running keeps me healthy and at peace and makes me sleep well.

I typed law briefs for one Iranian lawyer; each page was worth 1 cent, and I type 20,000 pages.

One important concept came to the top of the pile; how many young American men never had a dad! They often said to me, "You have a dad?" These man faces were full of anger and fear!

Now, I have experienced being wealthy, learning more about the working classes and the poor. Additionally, I learn about the foreigner and how they traded goods over sea. Some of the inmates collected 157 stamps from around the world. I could write a whole book about this experience; because many of you have no known idea what prison life is; prison life really only in the mind. Many of you are in prison from trauma, anger, stress, lonely, hurt, ashamed, and wounded and diseases; prison robe you (us) of freedoms.

Freedoms to think and to do! Many of us do note what could be. My biggest fear of prison was watching many inmates come back, because they were never changed by the process; because it's easy to do nothing. Only the personal activities that make you happy using the time up productively and do not think about the outside world. I took a class in art. I studied real estate and how to run an import/ export international business. I taught public speaking classes to an inmate from many different countries. I exercised six days one hour stationary bike after dinner. One night a week I played bass or piano in a band. Sunday was my weight day, 125 pulls ups in

12s, and pumped some heavy weights on the legs. Breakfast on egg days was different; they had eggs; sunny side, or hard egg, two lines. Sunday morning was an egg day. I precooked a bag of white rice in the microwave to add to my eggs in the chow area. I would be very hungry after work outs so I always eat a large breakfast.

Inmate attitude changes two different times. Fights occurred when stresses would mount. The young men would pace like a pack of wild dogs. Why the prison personnel didn't see it. I do not know? One episode occurred one evening, and I had gone to the chapel for medication with a friend. When we walked out the Chapel, he and I looked at each other. Since there was an eerie feeling in the air; we turned around and quickly went back into the Chapel. Just then the alarm went off—city fights in the yard.

Trauma—why does the public like to experience it? One evening a fight started near one of the units in the yard, the chow hall emptied. Not me I went back trough the chow line for more food.

The "runners high" was the experience while playing squish. I had become healthy, and I had good speed from riding the stationary bike. I was playing squish with a friend, and he hit one ball that looked as if I could not get it. However, with quick speed and to facilitate this magical moment I reached for the ball and got it. This moment was in split time I could see and feel the magic moment, just like it was in slow motion. My squish partner could not believe it! I had this type of experience 2 more time; living in the moment; I was out of the mind prison experience.

Incarcerated, this day I was feeling kind a ruff (depressed) (lack of energy). Consequently, I went to the gym, because I am addicted to exercise. I got on the treadmill, because the yard was closed. I started running at a good pace, and then turned it up to 5-minute mile. My legs were moving faster than I had ever run. I ran for more than three minutes at that pace and when I slowed down and noticed how tremendous, I felt, now. Exercising is fun and it is worth time, because it cleans up mind.

Inmate clerk, my job description, which means I answer the phone and type letter. First, I worked as a clerk on the inside, then after nine mouths I was giving a clerk job outside the gate/fence. Working on the outside started, after breakfast; go to the gate and get to check out and 4 pm checked in. While working outside the gate, I could drive a pick-up truck, when needed. At one location, there was a wood pile beside one of the metal buildings. The foreman/inmate Workers load up tools/materials. Then they went to campus houses, where they work on roof's homes. I would sit on the wood piles for hours. I learned about the layering of time in natural activity. What I learned to understand was at 7:30 certain insects, small animals and birds come from out of the bushes and woods and then returned there. The 8 am groups included insects, butterflies, and red wing black birds. After the first two groups, came the 9 am group with flies, and crows. I beyond doubt enjoy every moment of this time with and in nature. Because time with nature, clears the mind and makes it peaceful; even in the most trying situations. In the end, Incarceration afforded me time to smell the roses. There are many roses in our lives, if you look for them. Our simple lives will be, for the most part, balanced. Then add the daily touch and living is worth it!

The Love Touch will help you smell the roses!

When I was released and started probation, they sent me to the west side of Detroit where I live in the house with other probation men. I could not drive and had to walk to the Sec. of State of Michigan and stand in line three different times, all to get my driver's license renewed. My job was in another town, and I had to get a ride with an inmate (not right to do here). Nevertheless, my boss allowed me to obtain drivers test and license. Other times I had to ride the city bus to get to other places.

The next three year is very different for educated man working as a pizza delivery person and then a chauffeur driving for Metro Car. Workers in these areas of business are described as scorpion personalities, because they need to eat and look out for themselves. Even so, they will cut our throat getting there. What I know is they know where all the good tippers live as well as all the good-paying locations. I was for sure that they did not want to share them with a new person. Why work so hard at winning when you can win more by being fair! Maybe not they think, but really The Love Touch could help here.

Hip replacement surgery occurred after falling down hurting my back on a farm porch delivering pizza. Six months later I had enormous pains on my left hip while entering the car. Then I walk with cane for two years until I do get disability insurance in order that I could have replacement surgery. When you do not have the right color insurance card, the service is different. Being highly educated allows me to have the understanding that all people in American are not treated the same.

Please think about how unfair health delivery is to the middle class and poor. I went into a medical supply store just before my hip surgery looking for a wheel chair. I ask about it and showed them my green insurance card. Shockingly, they hurried me out the store not answering my questions and/or needs. They wanted no part of green card insurance!

Post operation was not hard; however, I itched from reaction to the bleach in the sheets. The whips and itching was harder to deal with than the actual surgery. They had me walking, the next day with a Walker. Five days of post operation care I walked with the Walker; then home from the hospital. I had to wear a brace in order that I would sit cross legged. The therapist came to exercise me and make sure I could get bath and cook for myself. Six-week post operation I was walking with a cane. Within 6 months, I was walking without the cane. The exercise sheet instruction stated that I should exercise

2 x a day. However, I worked out 4 xs and twice a day. I walked 5 miles a day for one ½ years. Bike riding added 40 miles/day. I have exercised all my life and enjoyed it. Therefore, exercising often is easy for me. In spite of this, healing has taken longer than I thought. So I added natural therapies at allow me to turn the corner. What I know and understand now is 100% healing takes a lot of work. Having hip surgery is work, and The Love Touch can help.

Life is full of wonderment with a purpose and gives us understanding if we embrace it. Since after the life's moment's passes it's too late to look for answers now; they have passed you by. That is why it is valuable to take time to look and see how important odd things are in our lives experience! Small events add up. Why do I know that, because without all the good and bad I have been through has something there? It is in the direction that adds value to my present life? Therefore, you or I could take what we have learned and cause a change in other people lives.

What did the garden tell me? I am warm and I have life's energy to make crops grow!

What did the farming tell me? If you work the ground and feed the stock, I will deliver grain, new knowledge, and trust and understand, learning to care about what happens; live stock, productions and self-wroth come.

What did Dad teach me? He taught me to communicate with my neighbors and care about them. Ultimately, teaching me to touch with love. He taught me the love Big Band Music.

What did mother teach me; to teacher, and to service others. Additional, she taught me to love the performing good music. Learn to facilitate Musical Bliss when play and practicing.

What did wood tell me? Wood is King of the Earth's elements that get used in so many places and products; houses, tables, chairs, decks, the cross, bury people, boat and so much more. Wood works with water to grow; wood is pliable and has many shapes that make our sitting more comfortable. Wood works with leather! Wood master pieces are used in all of our lives. Wood smells when it burns in the fire pieces and looks natural. The cross was making out of woods!

What did working at the gas station tell me? Work hard to be on time, keep the customer happy. Gambling doesn't pay!

What did University tell me? Learning is fun and it adds to your overall strengths of character; I learned to live with all types of people.

What did the Industrial Clinic tell you? Rock bottom Clinic Medicine concepts and working with patience's!

What did Medical School tell you? Believe in ourselves and service others; stop, look and listen!

What did ER tell you? There are lots of snakes (daily happening) out there, but they can be mastered in time!

What did incarceration tell you? Don't come back, there a lot of hurting men out there, who have never had a dad! They are part of the wounded living; The Love Touch can help!

What did one of my daughters tell me? She was born with nerd gene! She loves to study and learn, too.

What did pizza tell me? Has a lot of patience and worker needed daily touch?

What did hip surgery tell you? I have learned art of the body healing through this experience. I have learned that you must work with it; give the body what it needs, and it will heal you!

What did all this together tell me? It's great to be alive; exciting to learn the important concepts of touch; sharing it with others will change our lives; be grateful for those who spent time with you. What could I learn and add to my life, to make me a better person? Who has been sympathetic and caring on the subject of my neighbor? To not at all be bored, because there is a lot to learn and understand!

What did the research on touch tell me? Daily touch is as important as breathing; come please read ahead and learn to be worthy of the change. All your questions about touch will be answered. And if they haven't been answered the 1st time read it again. For these concepts are simple, and you must experience it; then you will be changed.

America (U.S.) Today!

The world's strongest military nation and wealthiest nation—America, however, we are the twenty-fourth nations on the earth according to the World Health Organization (WHO). Accordingly, the BBC states that Japan is the number one nation in the world. The United States—spends more on healthcare that does any other country. American has the great pharmacology. Pharmacology works with how drugs interact within biological systems to affect the function, while pharmacy is a medical science concerned with the safe and effective use of medicines. We must open our minds to the natural healing therapies that could make us healthiest so let's use daily touch? What about lifestyles change and make America a healthier and affect the cost of medical care and the business world! Add the two healthcare concepts together and then watch a synergistic health event.

While we look at these results, we recognize that Pharmacology and Healthcare do not take into contemplation the human circumstances of life-style. We should treat the family; not just the individual? We can have and examined and lab test, then prescribed medicine after being diagnosis. On the contrary, let us understand today's stresses and family daily problems? Gas price going up; costs of living is up; costs of medicines are up. One stress after can cause cancer, diabetes, stroke and/or heartache! The most-recent research has shown that only 35 percent of pharmaceutical medicines are taken as medicine and 50 percent of all prescriptions are not even taken. Historically, we react to physicians and taken medicine according to our family's experience. The Love Touch wants to help rid American families of the evils of improper family histories; stress and disease by introduce daily touch.

The irony of the high spending in Healthcare and Pharmacology hasn't proven efficient at translating expenditure into successful health. While the United States "is the most technologically and pharmaceutical advanced country in the world, some more than 40 million of their populations are without health insurance. This population has problems accessing healthcare and are leading in unhealthy sedentary lifestyles." All life styles need daily touch, water and exercise!

I have a friend whose family has adopted two children from foreign countries; their son came from Russian, where two-three child-care works were responsible for raising hundreds of children. Their daughter came from Korea, where two child care-workers were provided per child. The son was a very stressful child, because he had not been touched or cared for like the daughter. The daughter wanted to be held and touched, while the son fought while eating; and taking his medicine and had real problems dealing with other children. The son has ADD and had to take medicine, and his sister was balanced and peaceful. When I had the parents touch the son's neck before give him medicine, he was easier to work with.

If you rub a baby's belly for seven to ten minutes during the day, the child will go to sleep faster and rest well.

All the problems related to health dilemmas, and diseases could improve with daily application of the love touch methods. These entire problems cause the same effect on people in our society-stress, depression, more diseases, cancer and unbalanced lives. Americans have 14 different connective tissue diseases that no other countries can identify. Why, because they do not have the healthy foods and live in much less stress. Therefore, simple daily touch to stressful people can cause a change and cause a change, now!

Dr. Christopher Murray, director of WHO (World Health Organization) Global Programmed on Evidence for Health Policy, said: "The position of the United States is one of the major surprises of the new rating system.

"Basically, you die earlier and spend more time disabled if you're an American rather than a member of most other advanced countries."

Why does the US rate so low? It is due to the very poor standard of health among some ethnic minorities and people, who live in the inner cities. Again, Family's stressful histories can have a positive effect when touched properly.

Coronary Vascular disease is number one. Coronary disease can always be reverse and/or prevented with proper education of diet and experience with the love touch. Research has proven that touch of a medical student allowed them to complete their daily work in a much shorter period time. More noteworthy is that they increase the performance of over-all project and life. What you can glean from these studies is the powerfulness of being focused on the work at hand, when touched daily. When our minds are clear, then we feel well about our afterward performance with positive changes. We will talk more about the important to touch and being focused.

An estimated 21 million Americans have diabetes. Another 41 million people have the pre-diabetic condition of elevated blood sugar, which places them at risk for developing the disease soon. The American Diabetes Association estimates the high cost of diabetes, to be at least $132 billion a year as of 2002. This includes such expenses as disability payments and lost days at work. This epidemic has come, because of our bad health habits and poor life-styles. Daily touch could help with chronic illness and the cost of healthcare.

Diabetes is the sixth most common cause of death in the United States. Would America's Big Business, Schools at all levels, and

Government Offices be extremely excited about better revenues and less insurance cost? Their Board members will think about giving large dividends and bonuses. Best of all Americans and America would function more affectingly. Thinking out of the box will improve are effects to the highest degree!

In many cases, the poor are unable to afford fresh foods that are both healthy and appealing. They are either handicapped by a lack of education on good nutrition. They are less likely to use the supermarkets in their neighborhood, but buy from the corner store or gas stations. They are weighted down with daily stresses, which include low wages, day to day worries, family problems, and lack of energy, because of poor nutrient. The Love Touch can reverse these negative states of mind and energy; by bring the touch for 15 minutes every day.

Others eat unhealthily or overeat because it is one of the few pleasures that are within their reach. The results are a substantially higher rate of obesity among the underprivileged and intercity whites and people of color. Yes, poor intercity people are lacking daily touch. In a given view of the fact that touches can be free. They can become wealthy in touch, become focused, and change their world.

In truth many of these pre-diabetic people lack good healthy habits; they just live in families that are negative, stressful and depressed. All these condition need touch! More people go to bed each night lonely. Because no one touch them and acted like they care. Touch those who need it and America would change. Touch has no barriers of social standards, color, nationality, religions, sex, education, disability and/or adults or children; we all need daily love touch.

The hard part in all this is not declaring what needs to change;
It's getting organized medicine to start supporting that change.

Let us pray that the powers of modern medicine would integrate Love Touch within it hollow chambers of healing.

In the 60' America's children were raised by flower children, which used drugs freely, partied often, went to war, became educated and freethinking. They were open-minded from the old-fashion family life. Where fathers went to work and mothers stayed at home, to take care of the home and children. When the man comes from work, the children ran to him for a large hug. Later, they could sit on his lap and read a story book. The Love Touch was a grand part of the old-fashion family. It hugs were given when you left and come home. Children of the 60s believe that they were born free. The Love Touch was not important or a part of their life's, but good foods, good times to dance and be alive; freedom!

American Children of 60s were a hippie, and they learned to eat a variety of fast food, which included French fries and chicken nuggets. These Children never learned how to eat fruits and vegetables. They forgot about home-cooked meal. American children had children who learned to eat fast food for school lunches. What happen to peanut butter and jelly sandwiches and cheese and crackers? Mothers or fathers while feeding the young child vegetables had unhappy expressions on their face. How is a child going to react? How can the child be happy and think healthy about those green foods when the food giver gives negative environments about what should be good food health? Touch Research has proven that touching the child nap of the neck or belly, while at rest will make the child fall asleep faster and rest well. Timely sleep is important to better health and affects the attitudes of us all! Having an overall peaceful life makes the training of eating foods easier.

Today, there are several cookbooks that how to puree foods like squash, oats, and spinach. Then these health foods are prepared in cookies, chicken nuggets, browns, and pan cakes. The American children love eating these dishes, while taught those vegetables are important foods for good health. Additionally, the cook books instruct the parents to place vegetables next to the pureed cooked dishes. This in the directions gives understanding that vegetables create valuable health. A synergistic effect occurs when you add healthy habits to the Love

Touch.

Ray Kroc, who started McDonald's had a vast understanding of the needs of children and recognized that kids' meals would bring them to McDonald's several times a week. The meals were only to satisfy the need of hunger and glorified the gift. Basically, this made the children content with the toy without considering healthy nutritional needs. This in addition made the parents happy for a little while. What did the poor continuous eating habit bring? Unhealthy, out of balance children, will become sickly and obese; are looking to diabetes in the future? American children are heading into a Diabetics Epidemic, because of the obesity in America. We are what we eat. The Love Touch can touch with fast food children with a proper touch that will make their obsessive eating habits change for the best health experience. A Research Psychologist touch's patience with bad habits and allows them to overcome their stressful patterns. The Love Touch can help unhealthy Habits!

American Schools were paid millions of dollars by large soda companies to place soda machine in grade and high schools in all 50 states. This indulgence causes obesity and unhealthy children. Today, they are removing these machines and changing the dietary requirements. American school systems are starting to add exercise programs to help relieve the obesity crises in America.

Often children over indulge, because of stress in the young lives. Many of us do not know or understand that stress, and depression can start in infancy. Children with anger depression before 2 years old will have a CAT scan of the brain that shows old people's brains anatomical look, as if they were—65-year-old, losing essential brain tissue that can never be replaced.

This is very sad; nevertheless, the Love Touch can help these children significantly!

Ray Kroc and other fast-food-companies are not the single cause of America's health problems. All of us need to speak out when extremes occur in society. We need moderation in all that we do and our lives will be much better. Stress and disease come with over doing. We all need balance in our busy lives. So let's add The Love Touch and make our lives better.

A 39-year-old man was talking about his unhealthy eating habits in the sweat room where I exercise. He stated that he eats only meat and potatoes and no vegetables or fruit. When he passed by me, his skin appeared muddy, aged, and unhealthy. Healthy skin comes from drinking water, and being touched daily. People who eat whole grain, fruits and vegetables make their skin shine and beautiful.

Jack where I exercise stated that he eats only fast food three times a day; because he is stressed. He recognized how unhealthy that was he was so he was sweating and working out daily. Unless he changes his eating habits, he, will stay imbalanced. Adding proper Love Touch would make his life more balance.

There are hundreds of unhealthy life styles that live without daily touch. Just think if we could touch half of them and 20 to 30 percent of them start feeling better about them. Yes, touch helps one recognized that they are a human being, too! One of the worst problems with unhealthy life-style is that anybody can treat themselves poorly. What about learning how to respect oneself. Respect yourself gets touched and feel alive.

Change

Education could teach proper touching of others and change our world! American School systems need touch education to dealing with hugs during school hours. Our world is full of perverts and sexual predators. I need to understand how touch properly fits into your busy lives. What is it that makes touch so important to our daily need?

The Love Touch allows people to understand that other people are a human being too! The problem with sex offenders and many of the human crimes is that they see others as only objects. Inanimate objects or possessions are not important to any of us. That is why The Love Touch needs to allow one to experience the powers of human need of touch and then no one could violate another person.

Americans who live stressful, depressed lives have very difficult life styles. Worry Life styles lead to sleepless nights, poor bowel habits, headaches, and body aches. Their troubled days are filled with pain and personal hurts. What if these people could be touched? Their life would change with sleep, healing moments, and quiet times. A peaceful life could come in order to be.

There are hundreds of web sites dedicated to relieving unhappy lives, stress, anxiety, and depression. Touch causes release of the powerful neurotransmitter Oxytocin that response in mil-sec. Significantly, Oxytocin functions to increasing trust and reducing fear in our emotion body. Cortisol, in contrast, is the stressed produced neurotransmitter that caused pain; headaches, muscle tension and body aches. Cortisol causes many more negative effects on the human body that causes disease.

Cortisol

While Cortisol is an essential and supportive part of the body's response to stress. It's all-important that the body's relaxation response to be activated so the body's functions can return to standard. Sadly, in our current high-stress culture, the body's stress response is activated so that functioning doesn't have a chance to return to be regular. Cortisol produces chronic stress.

Higher and more prolonged levels of Cortisol in the bloodstream (like those associated with chronic stress) have been shown to have negative effects, such as:

- Impaired cognitive performance
- Suppressed thyroid function
- Blood sugar imbalances such as hyperglycemia
- Decreased bone density
- Decrease in muscle tissue
- Higher blood pressure

Lowered immunity and inflammatory responses in the body, as well as other health consequences

- Increased abdominal fat, associated with a greater amount of health problems. Some of the health problems associated with increased stomach fat causes heart attacks, strokes, the development of, higher levels of "bad" cholesterol (LDL) and lower levels of "good" cholesterol (HDL). Elevated cholesterol's can lead to additional health problems!

To keep Cortisol levels healthy and under control, the body's relaxation response should be activated daily. You can make lifestyle changes by keeping your body from reacting to stress in the first place. The Love Touch can be supportive relax the body and mind, aiding the body in maintaining healthy Cortisol levels.

Oxytocin

Oxytocin (Greek: "quick birth") is a mammalian hormone that also acts as a neurotransmitter in the brain. The most important stimulus for release of hypothalamic Oxytocin is initiated by physical touch.

The act of nursing or touch is relayed within a few milliseconds to the brain via a spinal reflex arc. These signals impinge on Oxytocin-secreting neurons, leading to release of Oxytocin.

In females, it is released in large amounts after distension of the cervix and vagina during labor, and after stimulation of the nipples, facilitating birth and breastfeeding, respectively. In humans, Oxytocin is released during orgasm in both sexes. In the brain, Oxytocin is implicated in social recognition and bonding, and might be involved in the formation of trust between people. Furthermore, Oxytocin has been known to affect the brain by regulating circadian homeostasis, such as a person's body temperature, activity level, and wakefulness. It is released through non—sexual physical contact, such as cuddling. It can cause feelings of warmth, being relaxed, and decrease stress. It is believed that Oxytocin is coupled with emotional feelings of love.

Which neurotransmitter would you want to have in your busy life Cortisol or Oxytocin? The Love Touch will teach you how to stimulate the largest organ in the body and get the positive result. Oxytocin will soften our stress, while Cortisol will drive up blood pressure and lead to more disease and even cancer.

Could you believe that a life full of Oxytocin could make your unbalanced life come alive?

The hard part in all this is not declaring what needs to change; it's getting organized medicine to start supporting that change.

Touch needs for humans? Over the last 15 years, I have met many men who are untouched, unloved by a Father or man within their developmental years of their family life. They would talk to me when they meet my dad or learn about him from me. Many would ask, "You had a dad"? Their faces were befuddled with lots of sorrow. These men are unable to feel the void or loneliness within their hurting hearts. They have problems with marriage and do not know how to treat their wife, and children, because they live without experience and/or proper example of manhood. These men and many families need the knowledge of Love Touch, and that would make their families and lives well. The Love Touch cannot take the place of a father; however, love touch can fill the hollowness and met the need of belonging.

Find the Love Touch? Watch happy families that hug each other and touch each other often. This is common in France, and many of the Arab countries. Then there are many other families that act like a pack of angry dogs! They get up every morning barking and biting always hurting each other feelings. Drinking alcohol makes it worse. Then add stress and money problems it gets even massy stress. What these families need is the Love Touch to aid in stress reduction barking and biting each other emotions.

What is the cost of Love Touch compare to allopathic health-care? In 1965, Open-Heart Surgery cost $6,500.00; today this Surgery averages $265,000.00. These Heart Surgery costs are about $258.500 dollars more because it takes close to 20 healthcare works for each major surgery. Buying the Love Touch and important touch is. Compare the cost of Open-Heart Surgery/ Doctor's office calls and/or additional cost prescription drugs. The knowledge of touch has been with us more than 5000 years, and our basic tribal needs have not changes. Our need of food, water, family, touch, social needs, and good sleep are important. All the rest comes from taste learned customs and/or ethnic traditions. I would not be telling you to forget your family doctor; however, what I am saying is touch is valuable to you and your doctor. Outstanding to know that being touched daily is as essential as breathing.

Pharmacy cost increases as well as the cost of new medicines. First, The Love Touch can affect positively all the diseases with diagnoses, surgery and medicine. Furthermore, remember that the Love Touch can prevent many diseases caused by stress and/or depression. If you had to group of treatment! Have a group that just gets doctor diagnosis, surgery, and/or medicines and the other group get Love Touch before a disease occurs and if a disease occurs and there will be different conclusions. The vital cost is wellness and quality of life. Living each moment in balance and working in good healthy habits with each day Love Touch could make a grand statement. How important touch is to our everyday lives?

Hope is a belief in an affirmative conclusion related to events and *circumstances* in one's life. Hope implies a certain amount of *perseverance* this believes that an optimistic outcome is possible even when there is some evidence, to the contrary. Beyond the fundamental definition, usage of the term *hope* follows some rudimentary patterns, which distinguish its usage from related terms: Hopefulness is somewhat different from optimism in that hope is an emotional state, whereas optimism is a conclusion reached through a deliberate thought pattern that leads to a positive attitude. However, hope and optimism both can be based in unrealistic belief, or fantasy. Hope is often the result of faith in that while hope is an emotion, faith carries a divinely inspired and informed form of positive belief. Hope is typically contrasted with despairs, but despair may also refer to a crisis of faith. Hence, when used in a religious context, hope carries a connotation being *aware* of spiritual truth. (In some religions, despair itself is considered to be a sin.

In Catholic theology, hope is one of the three teleology vicious (faith, hope, and charity), which are spiritual gifts of God. In contrast to the above, it is not a physical emotion but a spiritual grace.

Hope is distinct from positive thinking, which refers to a therapeutic or systematic process used in psychology for reversing pessimism.

The term false *hope* refers to a hope based entirely around a fantasy or an extremely unlikely outcome. Examples of hopes include hoping to get rich, hoping for someone to be cured of a disease, hoping to be done with a term paper, or hoping that a person has reciprocal feelings of love.

Hope was personified in Greek mythology as Elpis. When Pandora opened Pandora's Box, she let out all the evils except one: hope. Apparently, the Greeks considered hope to be as dangerous as all the world's evils. However, without hope to accompany all their troubles, humanity was filled with despair. It was a great relief when Pandora revisited her box and let out hope as well.

It may be worthy to note that in the story, hope is represented as weakly leaving the box but is, in effect, far more potent than any of the major evils.

Hope is passive in the sense of a wish or a prayer-or active as a plan or idea, often against the popular belief, with persistent, personal action to execute the plan or prove the idea. Consider a prisoner of war who never gives up hope for escape and, against the odds, plans and accomplishes this. By contrast, consider another prisoner who simply wishes or pleads for freedom, or another who gives up all hope of freedom.

Martin Seligman in his book *Learned Optimism* strongly criticizes the role of churches in the promotion of the idea that the individual has little chance or hope of affecting his or her life. He acknowledges that the social and educational conditions, such as serfdom and the caste system weighed heavily against the freedom of individuals to change the cultural circumstances of their lives. Almost as if to avoid the criticism, in his book *"What You Can Change and What You Can't."* He is careful to outline the extent that multitude can hold out hope for personal action to change some of the things that affect their lives.

In Human, All Too Humans, philosophers Friedrich Nietzsche had this to say about hope:

Hope. Pandora brought the jar with the evils and opened it. It was the gods' gift to man, on the outside a beautiful, enticing gift, called the "lucky jar." Then all the evils, those lively, winged beings, flew out of it. Since, they roam around and do harm to men by day and night. One single evil had not yet slipped out of the jar. As Zeus had wished, Pandora slammed the top-down, and it remained inside. So now man has the lucky jar in his house forever and thinks the world of the treasure. It is at his service; he reaches for it when he fancies it. For he does not know that jar which Pandora brought was the jar of evils, and he takes the remaining evil for the greatest worldly good-it is hope, for Zeus did not want man to throw his life away, no matter how much evils might torment him, but rather to go on letting himself be tormented anew. To that end, he gives man hope. In truth, it is the most evils because it prolongs men torment.

William James strongly promoted the idea that prayer (related to but different as hope) had a strong, positive effect for individual good in someone's lives. More recently, psychologist Anthony Scioli (2006) has developed an integrative theory of hope that consists of four elements: attachment, mastery, survival, and spirituality. This approach incorporates contributions from psychology, anthropology, philosophy and theology as well as classical and contemporary literature and the arts.

In some faiths and religions of the world, hope plays a very important role. Buddhists and Muslims, for instance, believe strongly in the concepts of free will and hope.

Patient health questions come, because they want to be healthy, to be cured, to be in balance; not just given pills and be told that they will live with their disease for the rest of your life? Patients want hope!

For this very reason, hope becomes the hall mark of all healing. Accepting hope doesn't come so freely. However, hope grasped will give understood. Ultimately, that is why hope is paramount to know, learn about and embrace. Hope helps us make good sense of any situation(s). When we hope, together great things can come to pass.

How that you understand how important hope is let use fasten hope together with The Love Touch, and the Human Spirit will come alive. This is what brotherly love is caring in a passionate way. Mother Theresa mastered these characteristics in her personal love touch with the untouchables. What great astonishment's come to the untouchables? Lonely, outcast, forgotten children and adults felt peaceful and cared about; that is what we all what to have simple need met. Now the positive synergistic energies of hope and love touch together they can move mountains; let's change our world, today.

Since a child, I have (always) lived in and long with hope. For ever and a day working in the direction of good at others; always giving the vision of hope along the way! When I was a child, I would lie on a wood pile and watch the Heavens for hours. Hope in life come from the wonderment that is always there and cloud work together with hope and belief! Spend some time there and you too will appreciate this beauty.

My Mother was a great organist and pianist, so I hear Classical and Christian music every day from my beginning life and after birth. Music was played on the piano every day, and I learn to turn the pages on the music sheet for my mother when she played organ concerts. It was very special to me, because music has been enormous phasing and movement in emotions that give expression of joys and hope. The master musicians understood life and the need for full expression of it in instrumentation! We will discuss music later, because it is important to our well-being and works well with The Love Touch.

America Today!

Those who regularly allow continuous destructive chatter of the brain [depression, anger, loneliness, everyday stress, life's issues] need to positive impute often. We must battle chatter and pessimistic/ stressful minds; all of us have daily choices! Hence give yourself permission to learn one fabulous secret of life "Hope"! Now, take your busy mind off daily problems and work diligently for wholeness, wellness/balance! You have these good choices! Working toward them is difficult! Our brain is the very fixable and new pathway can be made. It takes courage to move forward, and stop the chatter and focus on newness of life!

What will it take to change? Accepting the spanking-new concept and applying them daily. By continuous working in the directions of the new concepts, great change will come. Be patience and believe that anything is possible. The Love Touch will help you get there because new the path will be made using these Love Touch techniques. Read on!

Change

Change is akin to moving into a brand-new house, starting an untested job, entering into a fresh relationship, the difficulties we face in embarking on a red-hot adventure often mask its potential for great joy and fulfillment. (Myss). Age has nothing to do with creativity, love, and or the enjoyment of life! Choose Life!

Illness or disease is very demanding and require your immediate attention. Eventual diseases cannot be ignored. When you're waking up it there, when brushing your teeth it is there, when you sit it is there, when you ride or drive in the car it is there, go to work, talk on the telephone, and a great deal more daily situation; but it is always there! We can discount its presents; however, it may come to haunt you at another time: especially at night. What we should never do is accommodate the pain. When we accommodate pain then we have lost hope and the body rebels with lots of sleep, irregular bowel habits; eventual the imbalance comes and makes our days miserable. The Love Touch will help these defective situations in the human body.

It hurts or pain tells us important effects about the human body. These signs and symptoms can be awakening to understand that it is time to change our attitude or even life-style. The power of choice is important, because often there are many good and/or positive options that are different and new. Knowledge is power! Their greater consciousness is always rewarding. Hence enormously different is the descent to self-pity. "Verb heals. Nouns don't" (Myss, 1997)

The most-recent research has shown that we can make fresh pathways in the brain, if when stimulated that you stop and think. Don't just responses when you are asked to do something . . . allow your powerful brain time to think . . . "Do I like the way I am responding to their question?" or "Do I want a new and/or better response?" So I think it though then give an appropriate contrasting response. When I work on refreshing responses than new pathways come. This is exciting and fresh and your emotions will feel different. You will like yourself and these new outlooks. In time the responses will be natural, and you will feel new-found self-balancing. Wow I cannot wait for you to change and be this new person!

We all have an inner self who is weak, sickly, and small in character or do we have strength, fortune, honor and self-respect. Most people are somewhere in between negative and positive.

Part of the dilemma of victim mentality is that it overlooks the ways in which we perpetuate and ultimately overcome what has to happen to us. Soon or the next time it comes you get caught up self-pity about past injury. It's natural! However, this is really bad for whom I want to be or become!

Consequence anger, depresses, more stress play havoc pursues, and results are not what we want. Yes, waiting is a choice, but why wait when acceptable health style choice moves us in the direction of the best! One day at a time; one day not bad things will happen. Let us work together for your respect!

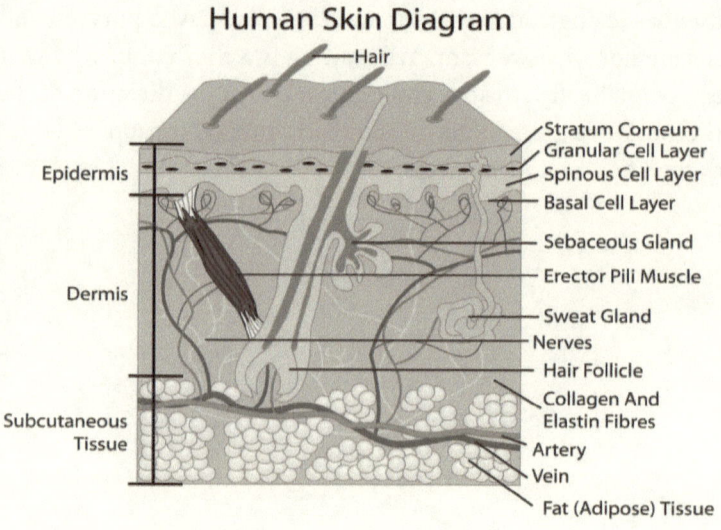

Human Skin Diagram

- Hair
- Epidermis
  - Stratum Corneum
  - Granular Cell Layer
  - Spinous Cell Layer
  - Basal Cell Layer
- Dermis
  - Sebaceous Gland
  - Erector Pili Muscle
  - Sweat Gland
  - Nerves
  - Hair Follicle
  - Collagen And Elastin Fibres
- Subcutaneous Tissue
  - Artery
  - Vein
  - Fat (Adipose) Tissue

Anatomy

Now we will learn some anatomy. This will help us to understand why The Love Touch is so important to good mental, physical, and spiritual health.

Skin:
We see the skin as merely as our exposed skin areas. However, "SKIN" houses the skeletal frame, muscles, connective tissue, circulation and vital organs. We should understand that pains over the skin are the tale-teller sign; a local response to cellular injury. We know and understand what caused chronic diseases and imbalance. We understand that internal inflammation will put you in danger of many connective tissue diseases. They are known as auto-immune diseases.

Diseases live in unhealthy bodies that are in acidosis. Dark sodas/pop has a ph of 1.2; this Acidosis is very acidic and a great danger to optimal health. Acidosis occurs when we eat any nitrates processed meats, excess sugar in sodas/pops, candies and much other starchy food; consuming copious amounts of antibiotics in meats; then unhealthy additives, and junk food. Unfortunately, what result is an acidosis tissue which causes human body multiple's disease quickly when you add stresses of today?

Cancer and other disease those Twenty years ago occurred in the 50-70-year-old patient. Notwithstanding, today it occurs in the 25-40 year an old patient. Stress and diet are the two most important habits that have affected the important shift in disease occur. We can affect changes and allow the body to work toward balance.

Skin is the largest' organ in the Human Body. Healthy skin is paramount to good health. Skin lay in three layers: epidermis, dermis, and subcutaneous fat. Our goal is to understand how important these layers play vital roles are that communicate an integrated signal to the brain. How our love touch will affect the brain, and its 200 chemical-physiological functions that communication took place in order to maintain our human bodies every minute of our day.

Skin is a membrane with protective functions. It presents a barrier to disease organisms. The skin is water proof; this enables a relatively fluid body to exist in the dry air. It likewise, permits the body to be immersed in fresh water without becoming swollen and in salt water without becoming shrunken.

When the skin becomes pigmented it protects the body from too much light. By sweating, the skin functions as an excretory organ. The skin contains nerve endings responsible for picking up stimuli that evoke many different types of sensation in consciousness (touch, pressure, heat, cold, and pain). For this reason, the skin is of the greatest importance of permitting man to adjust to his environment.

Each square inch of skin is composed of 19 million cells, which includes connective tissues, 625 glands for sweat, and 90 oil glands.

Nineteen feet of intricately woven blood vessels serve the square-inch area, along with 19,000 nerve cells.

Humans shed around 600,000 particles of skin every hour . . . about 1.5 pounds a year. By 70 years of age, an average person will have lost 105 pounds of skin. Human beings shed and re-grow outer skin cells about every 27 days, almost 1,000 new skins in a lifetime.

The average adult has 21 square feet of skin (about the size of a shower curtain) containing about 300 million skin cells.

On average, each square half-inch of skin contains: 10 hairs, 15 sebaceous (oil) glands, and 100 sweat glands.

The skin on the palms and soles of the feet are 10 times thicker than the skin on the face, and five times thicker than the skin on the rest of the body. The skin is thinnest on the lips and around the eyes.

Skin in total average-size person weights about 8 pounds.

Each square inch of human skin consists of 19 million cells, 19 feet of blood vessels, and 19,000 sensory cells.

There are 45 miles of nerves in the skin of a human being. Additional structures those are keys to our very complex protoplasm: Sebaceous, or oil glands (A) lubricate skin and help water preserves. A hair follicles (B) nerve sends impulses to the brain and gives skin its exquisite sensitiveness. Eccrine glands (C) produce to sweat this cools the body, and apocrine glands, (D) produce secretions that play a critical role in sexual attraction and produce secretions that play an essential role in the sexual attraction and simpler.

A Pacinian corpuscle (E) is sensory nerves that relay tactile information to the brain's hypothalamus, which records temperature and pressure. Capillaries, smallest blood vessels in the body; one red cell passes through the capillaries single filled (F), shuttle nutrients to the upper most layers of the dermis and epidermis then carry off waste produced by cell metabolism, and help release body heat.

An acne bacterium, which does its work in the hair follicles, creates acne by clogged oil glands.

Immune system, Langerhans cell, attack cancerous cells in addition to pathogens that penetrate the skin. When we exercise, live in stress, or skin temperature increases beads of sweat form on the skin the body; adjusting and working toward normality.

Epidermis the outer layer of the skin is our protection and covering by the stratum corneum, and it consisted of 15 to 40 layers of corneocytes. These flattened skin cells are layered with keratin/fatty liquid that acts as a protective barrier to prevent water loss. Keratinocytes is the building blocks of the epidermis product's keratin. Melanocyte produces pigment melanin, which protects the skin from UV radiation. Langerhans cells search for invading pathogens; therefore, they protect us from harm. Nerve's cells relay messages to receptors in the brain that recognizes patterns of sensations.

The body is very complex unit of tissue, cells and organs; however simple neurological changes with the touch will affect the over-all change for good health. We all want that!

Fat cells, which serve as cushioning, are more abundant; and there is a galactic network of capillaries, which connect to the veins and arteries. The palm has a greater number of large, sweat glands and has no hair or sebaceous glands. Sebaceous glands are present on the back of the hand. The palm' especially at the tips of the fingers has a net work of ridges called dermatoglyphics, which formed the fingerprints.

The Skeleton consists of 206 bones. Cartilage connects and supports them, and ligaments bind them together; this is a fine art. Let's continue bones are long, short, or fat, and compact or spongy, depending on the configuration. Their functions are to provide attachments for muscles and to act as levers for muscle's movement. Additionally, the skeleton protects vital organs and is housing of the bone marrow where blood cells are formed and stored there.

Muscle contracted is the force behind all body movements. Smooth, or involuntary, muscles regulate passages through internal organs and move substances through them. Striated or voluntary muscles move arms and legs, head and face, cavity walls, bone and skin areas. Cardiac muscle, which moves the heart, is also striated but involuntary. The muscular system is about 40% of the body's weight and uses 60% of the body's supply of oxygen and nourishment.

The more than 600 voluntary muscles in the body are connected to tendons than two bones. Muscles are described by functions. A mover causes an action; its antagonist produces the opposite action; a fixation holds a position.

Messages to the brain
The term touch includes several tactile senses: pressure, pain, temperature, and muscle movement. Many sensory receptors at different levels in the skin are responsible for conveying the nerve signals from thermal, mechanical, chemical and electrical stimuli. Meissner's corpuscles, located between the epidermis and the dermis on the hairless parts of the body-fingertips, palms, and soles of the feet, tongue, and sexual organs. These areas of the body respond to the lightest form of stimulation. The Pacinian corpuscles, located near the joints and deep tissues and in the genitals and mammary glands, respond to pressure, vibrations and high—frequency sounds. Merkel's disks, located just beneath the skin, respond to constant pressure. Ruffini endings, located deep in skin, can also register pressure and temperature.

Information from touch-sensitive nerve cells eventually crosses the sensory cortex to the opposite side of the brain where it is identified and response is given. The space required by the cortex is related to the size of the body parts. The nerve density areas with more nerve endings are fingertips, lips and genitals. They require more space in the cortex than the back, which has fewer nerve endings (fig. 1). Cortical nerve cells are highly specialized: some will respond only to stroking the surface of a body part in one single direction, other's response to stroking at a specific frequency. Those areas of the body with a high density of nerve endings are most sensitive to pain.

Neurotransmitters are the chemicals which account for the transmission of signals from one neuron to the next across synapses. They are also found at the axon endings of motor neurons, where they stimulate the muscle fibers to contract. And they and their close relatives are produced by the pituitary glands and the adrenal glands.

Neurotransmitters are a new and exciting field, because Wall Street, advertisers, psychology, as well as modern medicine wanted to know how our emotions work. Emotions control our heart and there are more pathways to the brain than brain to heart. The heart emotions can be felt 5 to 6 feet outside the human body. Often, we can feel the joy, and happiness in other being. Drugs can block neurotransmitters this important to treat disease as well as improve on other areas of illness. Because neurotransmitters are exiting, we well talk about them at another time.

Modalities that affect the skin.
Because the Human skin is so authentic and has special characteristics modalities well give us a better understands of wonderful the largest organ in the body is.

Epsom Salt
Before Wrestlers, contest junior high is trained, early in their athletic life, to soak in a bath tub of Epsom salt, four lbs; Epsom salt. Epson salt (Magnesium Sulfate) is a stringent, and it acts as an osmoality principal. Osmoality act pulls excess water out of the skin; the skin then cannot be used to pull down the wrestler during a match. The skin is a semi—permeable membrane; this allows proper materials

in fluids to be absorbed. The Epson Salt removes excess water from the skin. The skin becomes taut this allows the wrestler to compete at their best and not let the challenger to grab or pull his lose skin.

Epson salt directions: For external use . . . as soaking solution ½ cups in a quart of water, and apply wet, with a towel, etc; as a bathing solution: 2 cups added to the bath water for a refreshing bath after strenuous exertion.

Continually, Epsom salt is being used to remove swelling in the body from strains, and springs, arthritis, and even fractures.

Epsom salt a unique compound used to treat Pre-Eclampsia. Pre-Eclampsia comes about during unbalanced pregnancy of high blood pressure Epsom is administered by I. V.; Epsom soaks are used as therapy in arthritic joints. Epsom in a glass of water functions in the G.I. tract, soaks the skin, and placed in the vascular systems IV. No other medicine can work in all three areas of the body systems with colossal success.

Patch's medicines
Modern medicine has pharmaceutical patches and many specific ointments that are used on definite areas of the skin to acquire the therapeutic blood levels. Workable therapeutic blood levels of medicines are attaining through the skin affect the target organ. Two good examples are: (1) Calcium patches replacement pill therapy is placed on the forearm to treat dematerialized bones . . . osteoporosis; (2) With vital success cardiac medicine uses medical patches on the wall of the chest.

Kinesthetic
Muscle strength can be examined by placing an unopened vitamin bottle on the chest at the mid-sternum area over the rudimentary thymus gland. T cells of Thymus gland are part of the immune system, and it is birth there. Next we have the person being tested to use their arm muscle's strength. You do this by having them flex

their arm muscles once with the vitamins on the chest and again flex without the bottle of vitamins on the chest. You will see dramatic strength changes with the vitamin detected through the skin and chest wall. This method can tell you the defenses of tested vitamins/herbs within the human body. Since the body, bear can be a response through skin and body what about just allow the skin to be the immense communicator whom it should be?

Manufactured NASA Wearable
Accordingly, NASA Research has allowed far-infrared wearable: socks, long under ware, comforters and more. Far-Infrared comes from the Ceramic Plates found on the underside of the Challenger belly. These Ceramic Plates protect the astronauts during re-enter. NASA Space Suits are manufactured out of Far Infrared materials, too. These unique commercial products allow lactic acid to be displaced from spastic muscles. Lactic acid is the waste product of working and/or stressed muscles. Lactic acid causes pain or acing. Lactic acid is believed responsible for depression, post-partum depression. Lactic acid is single most active toxins in the human body that cause sprain, strain, muscle spasms and pain and more pain. Far infrared causes the water to vibrate within the muscle cells, water then moves waste like lactic acid out of the cells and many other unwanted products of metabolism. Exchanging toxin waste with nutriments, water, and oxygenated bloods is important to good health.

Magnetic products
Magnetic products use a measure of goass to describe the energy in these unique products. These products are worn on those areas of pain, aches, strain, and springs. These products give balance, and some relieve from discomfort. When you visit open rivers, ocean or woods after living in the city for a long time you feel peaceful, happiness and full of joy. This is because there are positive ions there. Additionally, we lose these growing positive ions when we drive cars, travel in planes, live around cement, cement and more cement. This harmful area in the big cities' blocks-out healthy nature

ions. Therefore, virulent areas give us additional stress. Magnetism can replace our toxic areas with cleaner cells. Several thousand years ago the earth gravity has twice as much. Healing with two x gravity would cause cuts to heal in hours not weeks like today. Some Researchers believe that they could make gravity plus chambers that cause increase gravity and sell healing. These positive energies can work together with The Love Touch and change our world. Positive ions come from pine trees, water areas and open lands!

Why the Love Touch?

We're all born with a remarkable need for daily touch. To thrive, newborns must be given to touch as much as food. Studies in orphanages and hospitals repeatedly tell us that infants deprived of skin contact lose weight, become ill and even die. We know that premature babies given periods of touch therapy gain weight faster, cry less, and show more signs of relaxed pulse, respiration rate and muscle tension.

Water
We will learn how to replenished water to allow the physiologic network to work at optimum.

Communication in the central nervous system
Neurons: Nervous tissue made up of live cells that receive, integrate and send out information. These are the basic links that permit communication within the nervous system. Just understand that million or trillions of neurons communicate with sensory neurons that then send a message to the motor neurons.

These high speed's connections that the skin depends on send the happy healthy message to the brain. The brain in concert with the neurons, muscles to move the human body. Movements include walking, running, standing, setting, dancing as well as other simple moves of the body. Particular movements like etching a spot on the back of your neck or adjusting your glasses allows us to function normally.

Etching is the form of pain that gives us an etching sensation. However, the neurons communicate to the brain as pain. Could this etch be telling something about your body? I even thought there may be fungus or skin abrasion there. Asian Medicine believes there could be underlying organ defiance or excess. Eastern medicine believes the largest organ in the human body skin can tell you much more that might be going on in the inside organs.

Additional hardware of the neurons is soma cells, and dendrites (trees) gather information and then communicated it to the brain. Between somas are axons, long thin fibers that send signals away from the soma to other neurons or muscles or glands.

Neuron impulses have electrochemical properties that transmit signals. These impulses can be read by the oscilloscope. The impulses become an action potential as voltage energy. Work muscle action and movement takes place. It researches to use these studies to learn more about the human body.

Research has proven that it takes more energy to relax then contract the muscle. Stress chemical Cortisol sends messages of hurt and pain to the neurons that cause chemical transmits to be tight . . . constricting muscle. Muscles tetanus assembles lactic the toxic chemical results of hard work as well as with strain/sprain and/or injury and accidents. Therefore, these toxins are build-up from lactic acid. Lactic acid causes pain. Pain medicines cannot stop toxic pain! Pains depending on where it is in the body can cause imbalance with the purpose of the chain react including the whole body. At what time situations of full body ache because life to be converted into stressful is unknown; however, you need The Love Touch.

The Bible state that, "We are fearfully and wonderful made." The human body must be taking care of as a whole being. The largest organ (skin) in our body can work in unison that will affect us positively. You will learn the small positive changes will cause significant results for your good.

Always, remember "Life is" an on-going experience. Learn to be an alive! Small steps can move mountains. It sometimes hurts and pains feel like sizable mountains. Let's learn to move these mammoth mountains of pain, stress and illness with The Love Touch.

Finally, when your brain receives to positive impute, which includes The Love Touch, and then strategies health building impulses will do their job by making new pathways. These impulses of hope are needed by our skin to communicate to the Brains support systems.

Attitude is important!
There might be easier to get the brain to believe that it can change imbalanced organ, tissues or supportive structures. However, for thousands of years much has been printed and/or researched for without this significant understanding the belief or good results could not come. The mind patterns of pain are learned. Pain is subjective pain for one person's pain is different for another person. New pain tolerances know how to occur over time.

I know of one lady, who believes that she could change her tortuous spine. I never saw this lady, only her boy friend who took still professional photos to document small changes in her spinal column over months. The most apparent changes on the photos were the appeared matted areas of new skin. This is large skin changed, and I believe that the skin will look normal in time. These professional photos showed me small changes, in the shape of her tortuous spine. Photos of these skin and spinal changes were taken over one and half years. She never when out or allowed outside influences to inter or interfere with her mind. She focused solely on healing and balance. Roughly, all of us do not have strength, time or drive to complete such long health goals. Just about all of us require exterior help; that why we have coaches, sparing partner, mentors, family and good friends. This exterior source help builds trust and adds strength to those in needs. One of the vital strengths of The Love Touch is building trust.

Mentors are important to our well being. One afternoon while at the Raisin River, Monroe, Michigan, I experienced a once in a life time mentor lessen. An Older Canadian Goose with a limp was leading a band 50 or move young Canadian Geese. They motored on a March towards the north side of Raisin River. The Young Geese March in unison while the old timer leads them over the waterfall into the brush and out of sight. This experience lives with me with grand delight in knowing how important life is, and that we should help each other March on. We cannot do it alone! We should help with knowledge. We should help with understanding. We should help with strengthen mine, body and soul. We are tribal people, and we need each other.

Hippos are fantastic social animals, which protect each other and take care of basic needs. The Love Touch in Hippo is always there. They are a great social animal, and we can learn from them. We must never forget that we are tribal, and The Love Touch reminds us of this important fact. The Love Touch was an historic factor in relationships within the tribes.

History of Massage, the oldest healing art
Massage may be the oldest and simplest form of medical care. Egyptian tomb paintings show people being massaged or having therapy. In eastern culture, massage has been practiced continually since ancient time. A Chinese book from 2700 B.C., The Yellow Emperor's Classic of Internal Medicine, recommend 'breathing exercises, massage of skin and flesh and exercises of hands and feet: they are especially used as the proper treatment for-complete paralysis, chills, and fever."

Greeks
It was one of the principal methods and relieves pain for the Greek and Roman Physician. Julius Caesar was said to have been given a daily massage to treat neuralgia.

"The Physician Must Be Experienced In Many Things," wrote Hippocrates, the father of Western medicine, in the 5th century B. C., "but assuredly in rubbing . . . for rubbing can bind a joint that is loose, and loosen a joint that is rigid."

Ayurveda, the traditional Indian system of medicine, places hug emphasis on the therapeutic benefits of massage with fragrant oils and spices. Aromatic therapies are practiced varying widely in India.

Doctors such as Amboise Pare, a 16Th-century physician to the French court, praised massage as a treatment for various ailments.

1785, C. E. Savary, a Frenchman, wrote about his experience receiving a massage in Egypt. "Perfectly massaged, one feels completely regenerated, and a feeling of extreme comfort pervades the whole system. The chest expands, and we breathe with leisure; the blood circulates with ease, and we have the sensation as if freed from a colossal load; we experience a suppleness and lightness 'until then unknown.

Swedish massage, the method most familiar to Westerners, was 1st practiced in the 19th century by a Swedish doctor, poet, and educator named Per Henrik Ling. His system was based on a study of gymnastics and physiology, and on techniques borrowed from China, Egypt, Greece, and Rome.

Physiotherapy, originally based on Ling's methods, was 1st practiced with the foundation in 1894 of the Society of Trained Masseurs. Notably, in Ancient Culture: Babylonian-Assyrian medicine: "If a man has cramps . . . place his head downwards and his feet (under him), manipulate his back with thumb, saying 'be good,' manipulate his arms 14 times, manipulate his head 14 times, rolling him on the ground . . .

During World War, I, patients suffering from nerve injury or shell shock was treated with massage. St. Thomas's Hospital, London, had a department of massage until 1934.

However, later new thoughts in medical technology and pharmacology eclipsed massage as physiotherapists began increasingly to favor electrical instruments over manual methods of stimulating the tissues.

Massage lost some of its value and prestige with the unsavory image created by "massage parlors." This image is fading as awareness of the value and a therapeutic property of the massage grows.

Germans Doctors use massage in their cardiac units with the grand result in hospital stay and treatments.

Modern Days
Now, Massage is used in intensive care units, for children, elderly people, babies in incubators, and patients with cancer, AIDS, heart attacks, or strokes. Most American hospices have some kind of bodywork therapy available, and it is offered in health centers, drug treatment clinics, and pain clinics.

The first perception input in life comes from the senses of touch while a baby is still in the womb. At that moment touch continues to be the primary means of learning about the world throughout infancy, well into childhood. Touch is critical for children's growth, development, and health, as well as for adults' physical and mental well-being. However, American society, claims Tiffany Field, is dangerously touch-deprived.

Premature child has a very tough time with life, and touch has been shown to increase survival dramatically, because touch makes them to look healthier and happier. Massaged preemies fare better than those in incubators on many counts; decreased stress hormones, temperature regulations, heart stability, sleep/alert cycles, and breathing regularity (Field,1998).

Families that infrequently allow the child to sit on their laps seldom hug or kiss them. Never shake a hand in the morning. It rarely gives them pats on the head for they have made an extraordinarily good job of a difficult task. (Watson, 1928).

Wilhelm Reich, the famed psychiatrist and psychoanalysis say, "It's not the psyche (mind), but the soma (body). Reich's successful psycho therapeutic approach to neuroses and psychoses was to hand touching the emotionally dysfunctional patient's muscular spasticity. Reich chose not to treat the psychological illness using the Freudian orthodox psychoanalytic approach of talking to the patient lying down on the couch. Reich proved that after hand touching the psychologically ill patient's muscular spasticity, the patient's cerebral repressions, inhibitions, anxieties, phobias, compulsions, obsessions, alcoholism, drug addictions, smoking addictions, gambling addictions, anorexia, bulimia, overeating, neuroses and psychoses, got better or disappeared.

We have all been given the Will to live! There is about 10% of the population that heard cancer or tumor from their doctor . . . as a death wish. Hope must not be misplaced, because without hope, the Will cannot fight on. I believe that the love touch can affect these hurting people positively.

Losing and Sweetman, write that AIDS patients feel isolated during their illness. They desperately need to be touched. Almost everyone, they know, physically distance themselves from AIDS patients because of the unscientific misconception of deadly contagions. "Without human contact, these AIDS patients give up faster and fall into enormous despair."

Maxwell Cade in London, England, in the 1970s: Using an electroencephalographic brainwave monitor, he found that the brainwave patterns of both healer and patient altered simultaneously as the healer started to concentrate.

It researches to have noted that women are attuned to the locations of touch, whereas men are attuned to the kind of touch that is practiced. Desmond Morris refers to us as a touch-starved society. Anne Gottlieb writes, "Frequent, loving physical contact with other human beings; cuddling, snuggling, stroking, hugging, holding hands, walking arm-in-arm around each other's shoulders, arms around the other's waist. All of us need it, and most of us probably don't get enough of it."

Dr. Stephen Thayer writes, "People, who touch arms, legs and other non-sexual body parts while communication tends to be more talkative, cheerful, independent and socially skilled than those who prefer a 'Hands-off' approach.

'Touchier' is fewer afraid, a smaller amount tense and a reduced amount of suspicious of others, while those who view touching as the intrusive or seductive end to be emotionally unstable an apprehensive, and usually have low self-esteem."

Science has uncovered many psychical studies that without touch, the Human bodies are not whole, but wounded. These wounds can be transformed and even healed when positively worked on over time! How do I know that I have a scare or wound? Scar or wounds have ugly, painful faces! Faces, especially the eyes can tell us what is in the heart. The spoken words give to use the pain of the heart too. Many unhappy days will produce anger, stress, depression, obesity, heart disease, cancer, neurosis and even psychosis.

Grounds for physical, social, and spiritual illness [imbalance]!

Wounds can have moods, feelings and actions that drive our obsessive personalities. Often, we do not know how to deal with these neurotic actions. The Love Touch will touch those stressful areas on the body and the body with give up those obsessive characters in good time. When the body hurts, so do the hurts of the brain. Remember the body; mind and spirit want to be whole.

In one recent case researches to have proven that those American children touch-deprived were brought up on carpeted floors lack valuable stimulating of the stomach muscle.

An early development stimulus of flooring materials has affected Americans live. One experiment took grown men and placed them on their belly-face down on flat slick or shiny surfaces, like those found in the kitchens in the 50s. What the study wanted to see the effects of development touches our emotions. Psychical studies get history of floor types patients were brought up on and noted that the sensory organs of the belly lacked early stimulation. After full consideration, research believed that without stimuli, we are continually stress, which results in depression and loneliness.

Touch deprived people many times lives of fear and the discomfort settles in the abdomen. Stress to the stomach muscle is isolated with the purpose of stays upset and trouble often. They live life with enormous neurosis and other abnormal physiological psyche. Men, who grow-up on non-carpeted floods couldn't lie on their stomach for minutes. Response was surprising when large adult cried with tremendous discomfort and ask to get up. If they were told to stay longer, they became anger and combative. When love touched child . . . floor lying response is comfortable. This is the normal response!

Memory cells occur because of traumas during work, exercise, play, and/or accidents. In other words, memory cells are caused by us and/or others. One good example is while playing baseball the ball is the throne to you, and you didn't see it coming so it hit you in the head, chest or shoulder or even back. We shake it off . . . "I am o.k.! "That didn't hurt me." However traumatic cell, acute inflammatory cell, will become the memory cell. Trauma is removed with exercise, massage, and/or therapy and nature medicine.

Even play one leg race, and you fall down and twist your back! You just got up with unpleasant discomfort . . . "I'll be o.k.! Yes, next day you can't walk, because you sciatic nerves hot from trauma. Pain running down the back of your leg and muscle pain makes it difficult to function ordinarily. Now and again, we seek treatment and therapies that allow us to function regularly within weeks and from time to time two or three months. Chronic back pain is common in America! How many of you have slept on the floor after lower-back pain?

Traumas Memory Cells happen over time and with age, they cause changes in our body shape and statue. Often, the body takes on a new . . . unbalanced look. I.e. backaches . . . cause Arthritis and other auto-immune disease. Dr. Oz stated on Oprah, "That after stress, surgery, we need physical treatment to help tone and balance our stressful lives." The Love Touch can help here, too.

Rolfing developed by biochemist and therapist Ida P. Rolf (1896-1979) used deep massage and "movement education." She authored several books on the relationship of form and structure in the Human body; these are used by Rolfing professionals Profound myofacia release "Memory Cell" in bodies that trauma and gravity have affected . . . crocked men and women from modern-day stress.

Rolfing research has established that we have "Memory Cells." Memory cell occurred when we have traumas in our muscles, tendons, ligaments. Memory cells hold metabolic fluids that need to be exchanged, or release. When Memory cells are opened by the touch or deep messages noteworthy changes can occur. Metabolic Toxins are released, exchanged then normality can occur. One celebrated example of these changes is sleep patterns. Often, these sleep changes allow active purging dreams. Sleep is important to healing and becoming balanced. The Rolfer works with our damaged body to help restore the memory, movement, and flexibility of the muscle.

Your eyes, in the park and can see a happy active human being. Looking on a couple sitting in a park, on a park bench, and he is rubbing her shoulders. Even just the eye beholding this can give the whole-body goose bumps. Memory Cells-even if it wasn't outwardly-touched. You have rubbed lotion on . . . therefore, pamper yourself. Furthermore, enjoy those goose bumps and "Bless" the lovers!

If we took the time to look and see the goodness around us; we would place great peaceful, pleasant thought in our brain.

These thought work for the good in us. So watch nature films, take walks in nature, site with relatives and friends. Learn to live peaceful with yourself and others.

The human body reacts to stress as sicknesses while a result of an inflammation response. Inflammation cause scaring that allow other forms of viral, bacterial, and even cancer to be noticeable. Auto-immune diseases occur because of inflammation.

Sugar is the number one food cause inflammation every time you use it scars and inflammation occur; just like stress. Fructose is the sugar used in a soft drink, because it is less expensive. Fructose does not act like sucrose when metabolized by the body. Fat cells from much faster with fructose, because it cannot be used really like sucrose.

A sick or inflamed body part always feels tense and rigid to palpation (examination by touch). Pain involved in inflammation varies with the individual. The tense and rigid areas of the body want the injured area too physiologically at rest and remain immobile. Then the inflamed area is less painful and works on healing itself. These tense and rigid areas of the body are known as spastic or episodic muscles. Sporadic muscles are involuntary and abnormal muscular contraction.

Pain house's inflammation, stimulates nerve's endings and causes hot pain. Chronic Pains cause muscle spasm that production lactic acid. Lactic acid is the muscle brake down a toxin. Symptoms most often include numbness, tingling and many other forms of dis-comforts.

Painful organs become dysfunctional out of balanced. Pain in the muscle or organ body is out of order; imbalanced. The human body is one complex system that works together as one wonderful unit. Therefore, I believe that The Love Touch can affect these abnormal changes, because the body wants to be well! It only takes a spark to get a fire going!

Scientific Proof that the skin communicates is meaningful and valuable information! Knowledge gives us understanding if we take the time to think about what is important and learn how it affects us for good.

Kirlian photography show that the energy emitted with lying on of hands. This energy is sent through the hands is can affect the balance of cell membranes, DNA and healthy living cells. Kirlian photography is definitive affecting changes in blood chemistry.

When the family member or good friend is sick . . . just simple strokes with hands can cause positive feeling. Other touches will help include, presses the head tenderly, rub the back, comforts and pets the sufferer, accordingly establishes a feeling of comfort and security. Domestic pets want and need to touch daily; cats arch their back when you touch their head, dogs wage their tails, pant and lick; horses need and appreciate currying and brushing.

Massage bed
Korean's beds have jade rollers and infra-reds heat. This bed rolls the back and neck and causes changes. Infra-red heat removes lactic acid.

When pains show relief, known hope and confidence follow with improvement.

Cold was a child were treated by Dad! Dad always rubbed my chest with Vicks vapor rub. Then he rubbed the bottoms of my feet with Vicks vapor rub and place warm socks on my feet. Dad gives me feelings of love, joy, and caring. These childhood experiences make me sleep well and in the morning I felt better. Just thinking about that experience warms my heart and inters my spirit. Little touches are important in our human life.

Touch has been referred to as the "mother of all senses" as it is the largest organ and also being the first sense to development in the embryo (Montagu, 1971) ultimately all the senses-sight, sound, taste, and smell are derived from it. It is important to know that the tactile system is the earliest sensory system to become functional (in the embryo) and may be the last to fade" (Fosshage, 2000) Touch remains the most important means of communication throughout our lives as well as holding the potential for use and misuse, for healing and for harm.

Caroline Myss, Ph.D. author of "Why People Don't Heal" believes that touch assist the unbalanced person to become more perceptive or simplify an attaining intuitive individual.

Field, a leading authority on touch and touch therapy, begins this accessible information with an overview of the sociology and anthropology of touching and the basic psycho-physical properties of touch. She reports recent research results on the value of touch therapies, such as massage therapy, for various conditions, including asthma, cancer, autism, and eating disorders. She emphasizes the need for a change in societal attitudes toward touching, particularly among those who work with children.

Tiffany Field is Director of the Touch Research Institutes at the University of Miami School Of Medicine.

How do we describe personal pain?

Subjective: def. referring to symptoms the patient knows and states he or he is experiencing but cannot be seen or ascertained by the examining physician.

Sensory Systems in the Skin: The Perception of pain is highly subjective and may be predisposed by mood, attention, personality and culture.

History tells us that we are not imaginatively new on the thoughts of touch; however, Americans have never been dealing with so stressed. Therefore, Americans need touch more than in ancient times! Stress comes from our activities and thoughts: electronics, work, family, social problems, terrors, sickness, depression, cancer, heart disease, diabetes and eventually death. Additional stresses to show up in our daily lives as headaches, body aches, dangerous bowel habits, sleepless nights, improper eating habits, nasty attitudes, fear, anger, loneliness and more. What about the stress from nature, it can cause high winds, elevated water, move house, destroy business and even families. We hear about stress every day on the news. This year has had California Fires, Ice storms in the plains and famous northeast, and floods many other American Communities. The world is much smaller, because of celebrated communication. I am not sure that this is good for stressful people.

Commanding rude energy, exhibited living in stress while not dealt with stresses immediately it builds the negative result. It actually builds inflammatory chemicals that affect our bodies; thus results are a disturbed body. "Oh, my pain helps me God! It is bad and it hurts! I would like it to go away!" Stress pains will go away, when we learn that pain is telling us something important our well being.

What pattern can I change in my life that will give me the good result?

When entire areas of skin are stimulus with the touch it causes the response. This touch is then interpreted very quickly by the person receiving the stimulus! Stimulus response is subjective in nature. Subjective-nest evolves from life experiences of touch, pain, and belief as seen in its similes form. Subjective learn process determent that we will be a response to pain and hurt.

Elementary perception of sight and sounds are not a passive process. We actively process incoming stimulation, selectively focusing on some aspects of that stimulation while ignoring others. Moreover, we impose organization on the stimuli that we pay attention to. These tendencies combine to make perception personalized and subjective. Studies have proven that people also tend to see what they want to see; see what they expect to see.

Thus, we clearly motives and expectations color our experiences. Overcoming subjectivity is what science is all about. Therefore, subjective characters can be changed by the power of choice and new beliefs. Potential include objectives that fuel the flames of hope!

We will learn that our modern society's Hi-technology, cell phones, scary/adventurous movies, copious tech messages, loud music, traffic jams; and stresses negative personality is killing us very slowly. Fifty years ago the black phone sat on the table, and ring went to someone was attempting to talk to you . . . not stress. Small amount of stress came while we were looking for a pay phone. Today people are talking or Text-messaging on their cell phone while driving on the super highway, shopping in the grocery/department stores, in the airplanes and while fishing on the water. Their slow inappropriate driving in the fast lane is hazardous. Cell phone talking and Text-messaging is suicidal to them and their fellow drivers. Research has shown us that the human being takes on the character of the electronic or machinery that it is connected with. Research has also said that answering a cellar phone, while the drive is like driving with three alcoholic drinks in you if you had to respond quickly.

Additional our thoughts are very important! Watch what you think about! Watch what you listen, too! Watch and think before you speak!

Since, the beginning of time, men have had healing touch. Nonetheless, research has shown the importance to the balanced life-style. Those deprived of touch have many physiological problems that could be comforted with daily touch t. Is it easily? No, however, it can be done if you work at it!

Your successes in healing or stopping pain are different every day, because healing is expediential. What do I mean? If one hundred treatments work, nevertheless, touch has a synergistic effect. Let me give you a short story. A lady who works will with trouble children. She took the cried baby to teach the other what to do with the baby acted out or cried. She talked to the baby while she rocked, prayed and rocked the baby for 1 and ½ hour. The next time it took only ½ hour. Then it only took ¼ hour. The fourth visit the child was place in the lady's arm, and the child went right to sleep. Don't you, I was sure hope this helps your understanding and gives you great hope towards balance and healing? Believe it and it will come to pass.

Mothers and Fathers have always been important to growth of a child; because the voices are contrary and touch is distant. Children require to positive impute of touch and sound in order to be healthy, happy and whole.

The Love Touch cannot do this alone we need alternative medicine and therapy personnel, which are trained professionally to help the unbalance and needy people. Some will want only professional people to work on them, and that is great. We are all in this together and working as one gives us power.

Today's Connections of the Love Touch: Massage!

What is Massage?; (derived from the French *massage* "friction of kneading," possibly from Arab *massa* "to touch, feel, handle" or from Latin *massa* "mass, dough"; in distinction, the ancient Greek word for massage itself was *anatripsis*, and the Latin was *frictio*) is the treatment and practice of manipulation of the soft body tissues with physical, functional, i.e. mechanical, medical/ therapeutic, and in some cases psychological purposes and goals.

Massage involves acting and manipulating the patient's body with pressure (structured, unstructured, stationary, and/or moving), tension, motion, or vibration done manually or with mechanical aids. Target tissues may include muscles, tendons, ligaments, skin, joints, or other connective tissue, as well as lymphatic vessels, and/ or organs of the gastrointestinal system. Massage can be useful to the hands, fingers, elbows, forearm, and feet. There are more than eighty different massage modalities. The most cited reasons for introducing massage were patient demand and perceived clinical effectiveness.

Peer-reviewed medical research has shown that the benefits of massage include pain relief, reduced trait anxiety and depression, and temporarily reduced blood pressure, heart rate, and state anxiety. Theories behind what massage might do include blocking pain signals to the brain (gate control theory), start the parasympathetic nervous system which may stimulate the release of endorphins and serotonin, preventing fibrosis or scar tissue, increasing the flow of lymph, and improving sleep but such effects are yet to be lifted up by well designed clinical studies.

Massage can be achieved by a professional Massage Practitioner, or by another health-care professional, such as Chiropractors, Osteopaths, Athletic trainers, and/or Physical Therapists. Massage therapists work in hospitals as allied health professionals, in nursing homes, sports and fitness facilities, spas, beauty salons, cruise ships, private offices, and travel to private residences or businesses. Contraindications to massage include deep-vein thrombosis, bleeding disorders or taking blood thinners such as Warfarin, damaged blood vessels, weakened bones from cancer, osteoporosis, or fractures, and fever.

Massage methods
Different specialized massage methods sorted in alphabetical order.

Acupressure

Ayurvedic Abhyanga massage
Ayurveda is a natural health care system originating in India more than 5000 years ago. It incorporates massage, yoga, meditation and herbal remedies. Ayurvedic Massage, also known as Abhyanga part of Panchakarma is usually performed by one or two therapists using a heated blend of herbal oils that are believed to be based on the body's dosha. The aim is to loosen the excess dosha through techniques such as kneading, rubbing, and squeezing. The feet are utilizing in chavutti thirummal, a specialized technique where the therapist suspends himself by a rope from the ceiling to apply extra pressure with his feet.

Barefoot:
Barefoot is a blend of Eastern barefoot techniques with Western manual therapy. Clients typically wear loose clothes while lying on a mat on the floor in supine, prone and side-lying positions with pillows or bolsters with no oil used. Because the therapist can apply a broad range of pressure with ease and does not have to strain.

Therefore, while being worked on more effort and concentration can be used to sense and manipulate tissue, and release fascia. Then search for attack trigger points, regardless of client's size or build. John Harris, who worked in the 1984 Olympics, developed this modality.

Bowen's therapy
Bowen's technique involves a rolling type movement over fascia, muscles, ligaments, tendons and joints. It is known not to involve deep or prolonged contact with muscle tissues as in most kinds of massage, but claims to relieve muscle tensions and strains as well as to restore normal lymphatic flow. It is established on practices developed by Australian Tom Bowen. [16]

Breema:
Breema bodywork is done on the floor with the recipient fully clothed. It consists of rhythmical and gentle leans and stretches. Fifty-minute sessions are common. There is also self—Breema exercises. The essence of Breema is articulated in the Nine Principles of Harmony.

Chair massage
Chair massage, also known as corporate massage typically lasts 10-25 minutes, and is achieved while fully clothed in a massage chair. Chair massage can be done anywhere. There are also chaired that robotically massage the client. i.e.

"Champie" (Indian Head Massage) in Mumbai, Maharashtra, India. Champissage

Champissage or (Indian head massage) has been worked with in India for centuries it combines massage with the more subtle form of chakra balancing. It is normally done by applying oil over the body. Additionally, Indian Head Massage is called 'champi' or Maalis. The word shampoo in English usage dates back to 1762, with the meaning "to massage". The word was a loan from Anglo-Indian shampoo, in turn from Hindi châmpo, urgent of châmpnâ, "to smear, knead the muscles, massage". It comes from Sanskrit/Hindi word "champâ", the flowers of the plant Michelia champaca which have traditionally been used to make fragrant hair-oil. It is often performed by the barber after a haircut on the head, shoulders, arms, and neck.

The term and service were commenced by a Bengali entrepreneur Sake Dean Mahomed, who opened a shampooing bath known as 'Mahomed's Indian Vapour Baths' in Brighton, England in 1759.

Craniosacral therapy
Craniosacral therapy is a gentle, hands-on method of evaluating the functioning of the craniosacral system, and is often mistakenly called to as a type of massage. It works through using the body's own self-correcting mechanisms rather than the application of physical force from the practitioner. When used by a massage practitioner, craniosacral therapy can usefully complement the massage treatment.

Deep tissue massage
Deep tissue techniques are, by and large, designed for more focused massage work. Working a specific joint, muscle or muscle group, the practitioner can access deeper layers of the soft tissue. Starting superficially and easing into the depth of the muscle slowly often allows more movements. If the pressure is deeply or quickly, the muscle may tighten to protect that area, and damage or inflammation may occur. Very little lubricant is applied as the pressure doesn't travel much over the skin.

The most commonly used 'tools' during massage may include, 3 and six fingers, reinforced fingers, knuckles, a flat elbow, opposing thumbs, the heel of the hand or foot, and the forearm. Profound tissue massage is similar to Myofacia Release.

Deep muscle therapy was fashioned by Therese Pfrimmer of Canada.

Esalen Massage
Esalen Massage was shaped by Charlotte Selver and works with gentle rocking of the body, passive joint exercises and deep structural work on the muscles and joints, together with an energetic balancing of the body.

Infant-massage
Shantala massage is an ancient Indian massage technique with a rhythmic character, given to massage babies and children. It was shaped into Western society by Dr. Frederique Leboyer, a French obstetrician.

Lomilomi:
Lomilomi is the traditional massage of Hawaii. As an indigenous practice, it varies by island and by family. The styles most known today are those of Auntie Margaret Machado of the island of Hawaii, Uncle Kalua Kaiahua of Maui and Oahu, and Kahu Abraham Kawaii of Kaua'i, who called his style Kahuna Bodywork. Other names given to massage performed in Hawaii are temple style, lomi lomi, lomi lomi nui, romi kapa rere, romi romi and ma-uri. Some of these styles may be traditional, and others may have been shaped by or created in modern times. The purported Lomilomi massage given by Barbra Streisand to Robert De Niro in "Meet the Fockers" was not an accurate representation of the style.

Medical massage
Massage used in the medical field includes Manual lymphatic drainage used for lymphedema [5] which can be used with the treatment of breast cancer. Carotid sinus massage can diagnose carotid sinus syncope and is sometimes useful for differentiating supraventricular tachycardia (SVT) from ventricular tachycardia. It, like the Valsalva maneuver, is a therapy for SVT. However, it is less effective than pharmaceutical management of SVT with verapamil or adenosine.

Myofacia release
Myofacia release refers to the manual massage technique for stretching the fascia and releasing bonds between, integument, and muscles with the goal of eliminating pain, increasing range of motion [equilibrioception]. Injuries, stress, trauma, overuse and poor posture can cause restriction to the fascia.

This is usually done by applying shear compression or tension in various directions, or by skin rolling. Myofacial release originators come from Physical Therapy and from Structural Integration (Rolfing); its current developers include John Barnes, Art Riggs, Michael Stanborough, Tom Myers, and Til Luchau. Dr. Oz had a Rolfer on Oprah.

Proprioceptive Neuromuscular Facilitation (PNF) and myofacial techniques are help to lengthen tight/ease muscles while fiber activation techniques are believed tone weak/ inhibited muscles.

Neuromuscular therapy
Neuromuscular Therapy (NMT) is used for pain relief. Perceived imbalances in Human position are evaluated initially through a postural assessment. These are addressed through systematic and site specific massage. In 1930 Dr. Stanley Leif, current practitioners at Paul St. John developed NMT.

Nihon Kaifuku Anma-Traditional Japanese massage
It introduced 1300 years ago, Anma is deep tissue work using no oils and is a kneading movements. Shiatsu massage grew out of this rich tradition.

Pregnancy massage
Doulas will often use massage to smoothen the labor process.

Reflexology massage

Pebble massages sandals from Dalian, Chi.

Reflexology, also called Foot zone therapy, is practiced without lotion, as the pressure points on the feet are stimulated by thumb and finger walking. Static pressure adds to this therapy. Foot massage practitioners believe that the ailment of an internal organ will be with the nerve ending on the sole of the foot. As pressure is put to the sole, theory holds that a healthy patient should not feel any strong pain. This theory is based on a perceived energetic flow of "meridians" in the body, also known as Chi.

Before the massage, the patient's feet are soaked in a foot bath for ten minutes, typically a solution of hot water and Chinese herbs. The practitioner rubs and massages the painful spots to break down rough spots and accumulated crystals, which have not been gathered. Based on this idea, some shoe liners are with pressure points to stimulate the soles of the feet.

Shiatsu

Shiatsu is a form of Japanese massage that uses thumb pressure and works along the same energy meridians as acupressure and incorporates stretching. While receiving Shiatsu, you are clothed while lying on a mat on the floor.

Soft tissue therapy

Treatment techniques include trigger point therapy, myofacial release, friction for adhesions between facial layers and muscles. Sustained finger pressure to lessen hypertonic, or tight, areas within muscle and fascia, active release therapies, and deep tissue massage are all derivatives of soft-tissue therapy. Different types of stretching include such as static stretching, dynamic stretching, and/or PNF stretching (proprioceptive neuromuscular facilitation).

Another form of Soft tissue therapy is muscle energy technique (MET) which uses reciprocal inhibition (RI) which is when the therapist uses a client's muscle to stretch the opposing muscle. The therapist takes the muscle that they are wishing to stretch to its full range of motion. The therapist gets the client to use the opposing muscle by moving away from the therapist. When the client relaxes the therapist moves the muscle force in a try to realign the muscle fibers.

Massage therapist working at a Triathlon in Fremantle, Western Australia, Australia. This is a common site at large sports events.

Sports massage
Muscle Energy Technique (MET) can be to the calf when the client is lying supine on the treatment couch. The therapist can place one hand on the tibia just below the knee to isolate the knee preventing it from moving. The other hand is placed around the heel so the therapist's forearm can be used to dorsiflex the foot. This can be used by sports massage therapists.

Stone massage
Heated stones were Egyptians, Native Americans and in Lomilomi massage. Smooth hot or cold stones, usually basalt or marble, are to massage the body. When heated stones are placed on the body muscles relax allowing the massage therapist to work deeper into the muscle, with healing acts. Energy medicine is sometimes incorporated into stone massage. Hot stones are placed along both sides of the spine, and on top of the torso. They are to heat the chakra or meridians centers.

Heated stones coated with oil are placed in the hands of the therapist delivering various massaging strokes.

Structural Integration
Rolfing, a method of Structural Integration, works with realigning the body structurally and human gait.

Swedish massage
These styles make the most of long, flowing strokes, often but not in the direction of the heart. There are six basic strokes: effleurage

from the French effleurer, 'to skim over', petrissage from the French pétrir, 'to knead', friction, tapotement, compression, and vibration. Petrissage is a kneading movement with the whole palm or finger tips, using wringing, skin rolling, compression, and/or lifting. Petrissage is applied vertically to the muscle tissue. Oil, cream, or lotion is on the skin to reduce friction and allow smooth strokes. Effleurage consists of long, flowing or gliding strokes, performed with open hands. In many massage sessions, effleurage is as the initial type of stroking, as it has a calming effect when performed slowly. Swedish massage has shown to be helpful in reducing pain, joint stiffness, and improving function in patients with osteoarthritis of the knee over eight weeks. [19]

Therapeutic touch (commonly shortened to "**TT**"), also known as **Non-Contact Therapeutic Touch** (NCTT), is an energy therapy which practitioners claim promotes healing and reduces pain and anxiety. Practitioners of therapeutic touch state that by placing their hands on, or near, a patient, they are able to detect and manipulate the patient's energy field one highly cited study, designed by nine-year-old Emily Rosa and published in the Journal of the American Medical Association found that practitioners of therapeutic touch could not detect the presence or absence of a hand placed a few inches above theirs when their vision was obstructed. Simon Singh and Edzard Ernst concluded in their 2008 book Trick or Treatment that "the energy field was probably nothing more than a figment in the imaginations of the healers."]

History
This style of massage is attributed to the Swedish fencing master and gymnastics teacher Per Henrik Ling (1776-1839). However, it was, in fact, the Dutch practitioner Johan Georg Mezger (1838-1909) who adopted the French names to denote the basic strokes. The term Swedish Movement System was to Swedish Massage System sometime during the second half of the 19th century. Ling's

system was the Swedish Movement System or Swedish Gymnastic Movement System.

He has become associated with Swedish massage.

The Aikikai foundation of the Japanese martial art Aikido incorporates a massage into their routine, in Slovenia.

Tai Ji/Tai Chi massage
Massage uses the natural principles of Yin and Yang to achieve balance in the energies of the body. Practitioners of Tai Ji believed that it uses Tao and deals with Qi blockages.

Thai massage
Known in Thailand as (Nuat phaen boran, IPA), meaning "ancient/traditional massage", Thai massage is also known as Thai ancient massage, traditional Thai massage, Thai yoga massage, yoga massage, Thai classical massage, Thai bodywork, passive yoga or help yoga. Thai massage in India based on Ayurveda and yoga, thereafter becoming popular in ancient Siam, now known as Thailand. It was the massage art brought over to Thailand by Shivago Komarpaj (Jivaka Kumarabhacca), a contemporary with Gautama Buddha 2500 years ago. The receiver is put into yoga positions during the course of the massage. In the northern style Chiang Mai, Thailand, there are a lot of stretching movements, unlike the southern style where acupressure is emphasized.

The massage recipient changes into loose, comfortable clothes and lies on a mat or firm mattress on the floor, then therapy begins. (It can be done solo or in a group of a dozen or so patients in the same large room.) The massage practitioner leans on the recipient's body using hands and usually straight forearms loceked at the elbow to apply firm rhythmic pressure. The massage follows the Sen Lines on the body-known as the similar to meridians or Channel (Chinese medicine) and Indian nadis. Legs and feet of the giver can fixate the body or limbs of the recipient. In other styles, hands fixate the body, while the feet do the massaging action. Oil is not in traditional Thai Massage. A full Thai massage session typically lasts two hours or more, and includes rhythmic pressing and stretching of the entire body. Often, this include pulling fingers, toes, ears, cracking the knuckles, walking on the recipient's back, and arching the recipients into bhujangasana or (cobra position).

There are a standard procedure and rhythm to this massage. In Thailand a two-hour massage might cost around 300 Thai baht (US $8 in 2005) depending on location (it may cost ten times more inside a five star hotel).

Germany Medicine incorporates massage into their hospital much more than Americans and other countries. Heart attached patient are even treated. Here Nuat phaen boran or Thai massage; side-lying position in Frankfurt, Germany.

Note: The traditional therapeutic practice of Thai massage should not the sexual service of the same name that is available in some hotels and brothels. Sometimes the traditional therapeutic Thai Massage, or ancient massage, is the "old lady massage", while the sexual practice, which has nothing to do with therapeutic traditional massage is called "young lady massage".

Traditional Chinese massage
Na is focusing on pushing, stretching and kneading the muscle.

Zhi Ya is similar to Tui Na massage except it focuses more on pinching and pressing at acupressure points. Both of these methods are based on principles from traditional Chinese medicine.

Trager Approach
The Trager Approach combines movement, massage and education.

Trigger point therapy
This is called pressure point massage. [5] A trigger point is an area of a muscle (about 50 cells) that may refer pain sensations to other parts of the body. Manual pressure is to these points. This work was founded by Dr. Janet G. Travell, U.S. President John F. Kennedy's physician and David Simons. This work can be integrated into other styles of massage therapy such as neuromuscular therapy (NMT) or Swedish.

Visceral manipulation
One form is Mayan abdominal massage which is in many countries in Latin America. This massage was by Don Elijio Panti and Dr. Rosita Arvigo of Peru.

Mantak Chia introduced a form of abdomen massage called Chi Nei Tsang, which he teaches, helps to "clears negative emotions" (in the form of "bad winds" or "sick winds") which gather near the navel.

Watsu
Watsu is the combination of hydrotherapy, and Shiatsu developed by Harold Dull in his time spent at Harbin Hot Springs near Middletown, California, USA. The work is done in skin temperature water with both the therapist and practitioner in the water, usually a pool which is between 3.5 ft to four ft. (100-120 cm) deep. The work entails many movements in the water and practitioners known that it's the activation of the energy lines derived from Shiatsu.

Associated methods
Many types of practices are massage and include Bodywork (alternative medicine), manual therapy, energy medicine, and breath-work. Other names for massage and related practices include hands-on work, body/somatic therapy, and somatic movement education. Body-mind integration techniques stress self-awareness and movement over physical manipulations by a practitioner. Therapies related to movement awareness/ educations are closer to

Dance and movement therapies. Massage can also have connections with the New Age movement and alternative medicine as well as by mainstream medical practitioners.

Beneficial [Helpful] effects
Massage is hindered from reaching the gold standard of scientific research, which includes placebo-controlled and double-blind clinical trials.[22] [23] Developing a "sham" manual therapy for massage would be difficult since even light touch massage could not be completely devoid of effects on the subject.[22] It would also be tricky to find a subject that would not notice that they were getting less of a massage, and it would blind the therapist.[22] Massage can employ randomized controlled trials, which are peer reviewed medical journals.[22] This type of study could increase the credibility of the profession because it displays that purported therapeutic effects are reproducible.[23]

Single dose effects
Pain relief: Relief from pain due to musculoskeletal injuries is a major benefit of massage In one study, cancer patient's self-reported symptomatic relief of pain.[24] [25] This study, did not include a known treatment or placebo control group so these effects may be due to the placebo effect or regression towards the mean. Massage can also relieve tension headaches. Acupressure or pressure point massage may be a beneficial to classic Swedish massage in relieving back pain.[26 On the other hand, a meta-study conducted by scientists at the University of Illinois at Urbana-Champaign failed to find a statistically significant reduction in pain immediately following treatment. [7]

State anxiety: Massage has been shown to reduce state anxiety, a transient measure of anxiety in a given situation. [7]

Blood pressure and heart rate: Massage has been shown to reduce blood pressure and heart rate as temporary effects. [7]

Attention: After massage, EEG patterns show enhanced performance and alertness on mathematical computations, with the effects perhaps by decreased stress hormones.

Other: Massage also stimulates the immune system [27] by increasing peripheral blood lymphocytes (PBLs). However, this immune system effect is only observed in aromatherapy massage, which includes sweet almond oil, lavender oil, cypress oil, and sweet marjoram oil? It is unclear whether this effect persists over the long term.

Multiple dose effects
Pain relief: Education and exercises with massage will help sub-acute, chronic, non-specific low back pain. [28] Furthermore, massage has been shown to reduce pain experienced in the days or weeks after treatment.

Trait anxiety: Massage has been shown to reduce trait anxiety, a person's general susceptibility to anxiety.

Depression: Massage has been shown to reduce sub-clinical depression.

Diseases: Massage, involving stretching, has been shown to help with spastic diplegia resulting from Cerebral palsy in a small pilot study. The researchers warn that these results should "be viewed with caution until a double-blind controlled trial can be conducted."

Massage has an effort to improve symptoms, disease progression, and quality of life in HIV patients; however, this treatment is not scientifically supported at this time.

Regulation
In the U.S.A. there are about 90,000 massage therapists. Training programs in the U.S. are typically 500-1000 hours in length, and can award a certificate, diploma, or degree depending on the particular

school. There are around 1,300 programs training massage therapists in the country and study will often include anatomy and physiology, kinesiology, massage techniques, first aid and CPR, business, ethical and legal issues, and hands-on-practice along with continuing education requirements if regulated. The Commission on Massage Therapy Accreditation (COMTA) is one of the organizations that works with massage schools in the U.S. 38 states and the District of Columbia require some type of licensing for massage therapists. [32] In the US, 32 states use the National Certification Board for Therapeutic Massage and Bodywork's certification program as a basis for granting licenses either by rule or statute. The National Board grants the designation Nationally Certified in Therapeutic Massage and Bodywork (NCTMB). There are two tests available and you can become certified through a portfolio process if you have equivalent training and experience. Between 10-20% of towns or counties regulate the profession. These local regulations can range from prohibition on opposite sex massage, fingerprinting and venereal checks from a doctor, to prohibition on house calls because of concern regarding the sale of sexual services.

In the U.S.A., the licensee is the highest level of regulation, and this restricts anyone without a license from practicing massage therapy or by calling themselves that protected their title. Certification allows only those who meet certain educational criteria to use the protected title and registration only requires a listing of therapists who apply and meet an educational requirement. [36]

In Canada only three provinces regulate massage therapy, they are British Columbia, Ontario, and Newfoundland and Labrador. The Canadian Massage Therapists Alliance (CMTA) has set a level of 2200 practice hours in Ontario, and Newfoundland and Labrador and 3000 hours in British Columbia. In India, massage therapy is certified by The Department of Ayurveda, Yoga & Naturopathy, Unani, Siddha and Homoeopathy (AYUSH) under the Ministry of Health and Family Welfare (India) in March of 1995.

Because the art and science of massage are a globally diverse phenomenon, different legal jurisdictions sometimes recognize and license individuals with titles. Examples are:

Registered Massage Therapist (RMT) Canada

Certified Massage Therapist (CMT) Licensed Massage Practitioner (LMP) Licensed Massage Therapist (LMT) Licensed Massage and Bodywork Therapist (LMBT) North Carolina

Prevalence in the United States
In 1997 there was an estimated 114 million visits to massage therapists in the US. Massage therapy is the most-used type of Complementary and alternative medicine in hospitals in the United States.

In 2003, 64 percent of families of a child with out of the ordinary health care needs reported that they use alternative therapies. These therapies included spiritual healing, massage, chiropractic, herbs and particular diets, homeopathy, self-hypnosis and other methods of complementary and alternative medicine. The used of an alternative therapy was to the child's condition and to the belief that it is or is not repairable. People state that they use massage because they believe that it relieves pain from musculoskeletal injuries and other causes of pain, reduces stress and enhances relaxation, rehabilitates sports injuries, decreases feelings of anxiety and depression, and increases general well being.

In a poll of 25-35 year olds 79% said they would like their health insurance plan to cover massage. Some of the companies that offer massage to their employees include Allstate, Best Buy, Cisco Systems, FedEx, Gannett, which runs (USA Today), General Electric, Hewlett-Packard, Home Depot, JC Penney, Kimberly-Clark, Texas Instruments and Yahoo. In 2006, Duke University Health System opened a center to integrate medical disciplines with CAM disciplines such as massage therapy and acupuncture. This trend was by Andrew Weil. There were 15,500 spas in the United States in 2007 with about a third of the visitors being men.

The number of visits rose from 91 million in 1999 to 136 million in 2003, generating revenue that equals $11 billion.

Research on the Benefits of Massage

Over the decades, many studies have investigated the impact of massage/touch on conditions and physiological processes. We invite you to familiarize yourself with this research. The following benefits have been shown conclusively, and more are discovered daily:

Massage is proven to:
- Strengthen the immune system
- Accelerate the elimination of metabolic by-products and toxins, such as lactic-acid build-up
- Relieve anxiety and depression
- Reduce elevated blood pressure
- Relieve insomnia and headaches
- Reduce stress and induce relaxation
- Improve musculature performance
- Increase mental alertness Improve circulation
- Restore energy
- Reduce feelings of isolation
- Relieve muscle tension and stiffness
- Free the body of pain caused by tension and low body fluid circulation

The Role of Love Touch in Infants

The Love Touch is generally a technique that combines tactile, kinesthetic stimulation performed in a purposeful, sequential application. The Love Touch technique for infants is much different from Love Touch for adults. It is not as much manipulative as it is communicative. It is a technique that allows parents to engage and relax their child in mutually pleasurable interaction.

It is not the Love Touch or the infant Love Touch instructor who Love Touch the infant/child-it is the parent/caregiver. Delicate interest in the love touch individuality is important to our understanding of touch. You, like the parent to these children become the primary source of interaction in the context of the infant's life. The dynamics of the love touch facilitate consciousness skills, person-person interaction, bonding and plutonic attachment, and the love touch's' person improved ability to read their cues.

Positive cues may include eye contact, changes in the color of skin, gaze at the persons face, making babbling or not that . . . it's too hard, or oh that feels really good. Negative cues may include pulling away, frowning or grimacing, turning the head away, speaking out, squirming, and others. You, the love touch person will learn what, when, where, how long and how much and it. They, the receiver don't know then together work it out. The focus of the love touch is not solely on the receiver, but on the reciprocal interaction between love touch partners. The Love Touch is not done to the love touch receiver; it is done with a receiver.

"Touching is the first communication a baby receives," says Frederick Leboyer, author of Loving Hands. "The first language of its development is through the skin."

Infants communicate through their bodies; you as an adult communicate with your body too. When you engage with the love touch person, you will begin to listen to the receiver; you listen to sound. You watch movements. You listen with your eyes, your ears and your heart. The love touch communication, nurtures the most important relationship the adults will ever have: the relationship between the love touch partners.

By using the Love Touch you will learn the art of listening, asking permission, communicating, interpreting and responding to cues.

For the mother of a child with cerebral palsy, infant massage has made a world of difference in her ability to open up a line of communication with her child. "My baby used to just be a baby," she said. "Now he is a baby, and he has a personality. Infant-massage gave him away to express himself-giggling or interacting in a dialogue when he had never been able to speak before."

The Benefits of Infant Massage by Elaine Fogel Schneider in the Psycho-social Domain Benefits to the infant of receiving Love Touch; these important benefits aids the infants as they become adults. Knowledge and understanding in these improvements will allow thought's adult who lacks any of the improvements below need the Love Touch. I.e. lacking good circulation is not health; if you lack strengths is not respectable.

It improves body awareness
It improves relaxation and release of accumulated stress
Stimulates circulation
It strengthens digestive, circulatory and gastrointestinal systems, which can lead to weight gain
It reduces discomfort from teething, congestion, gas, colic and emotional stress
It improves muscle tone coordination
It increases elimination, circulation and respiration
It improves sleep patterns
It increases hormonal function
Benefits to the parent of giving massage; The Love Touch person will receive much of the same good benefits.
It improves sense of well-being Reduces blood pressure Reduces stress
It improves overall health

Wouldn't it be great to know by doing the love touch that you will get better and better? Mother Theresa and Dr. Livingston learn as they treated the needy and who are ill they received the greatest reward. Peace of Mind and copious blessing

What Does Massage Really Do?

Physical Level:
Deep relaxation and stress reduction Relief of muscle tension and stiffness Reduced muscle spasm and tension
Relief from entrapment of nerves in muscle greater joint flexibility and range of motion increased ease and efficiency of movement promoted deeper and easier breathing
Better circulation of both blood and lymph fluids
Reduced blood pressure
Relief of tension-related or eye-strain headaches
Healthier, better nourished skin
Improved posture
Faster healing from pulled muscles and sprained ligaments
Reduces pain, swelling, and formation of scar tissue following injury
General health maintenance

Mental Level:
Relaxed state of alertness
      Reduced mental stress: a calmer mind
Greater ability to monitor stress signals and respond appropriately
Increased capability for clearer thinking

Emotional Level: Feeling of well-being Reduced levels of anxiety
Increased awareness of mind-body connection
Enhanced self image
      A sense of being unified and in harmony

Stress and the Body
We experience all of life through the physical reality of our bodies. Our pleasures and pains, the ups and downs of daily life affect the body profoundly, often in ways we're not aware of. Stress is more than a household word these days-it's something everyone feels to one degree or another. Let's take a look at the mechanics of stress and the role the love touch can play in stress management.

Understanding the Stress Response
Stress is an unconscious and automatic reaction to anything and everything we believe may be threatening to us; some stresses are not seen as stress, however, affect your body negatively. In the stress response, the human body is primed for "fight or flight" by signal that carried by the sympathetic branch of the nervous system. Whether we are confronted by a mugger in the street or find ourselves in a long line at the bank or a short lunch hour, the effects are the same, impacting all levels-physical, mental and emotional.

We are full readiness as our body tenses, muscles alert, and our breathing gets shallower and more rapid. You have stimulated the Para-sympathetic system. Without delay comes the full effect increase in heart rate, blood pressure and adrenaline production, with a corresponding decrease in blood flow to the extremities, digestive function, and immune system activity. Many Americans live stressful most of the day; this is very dangerous to our health. The Love Touch will make these vicious unsafe cycles normal.

Ideally, this defensive reaction will subside once the situation has resolved, allowing our body to return to its normal state of affairs. Still, we do not resolve the issue so the stress remains. I learn the hard way that stress is internal. Often working out helps remove stress. Nevertheless, work out only removes physical intention but not the neurological/chemical. Effects on organs, tissue and balance are dynamic. The Love Touch will affect is at the neurological/ chemical level, and if you add visualization and positive self-talk new pathway can form.

Learning and understand that sometimes rest helps the stress process. We in due course want to believe. However, without some improvement or results . . . we don't believe that they finally have excellent health is at the door!

Nevertheless, a person who is frequently under stress influences will tend to remain locked into a pattern of worry response, unable to relax or let go. Cortisol and Homocytine levels increase and cause heart disease. These chemical patterns are additionally are damaging to the body balance; as unbalance escalates, it ultimately leads to inflammation/disease, pain discomfort, and is a contributing factor in most chronic disease processes.

Pain tells us important signs and information about our internal human body. Often, we take medicine, sleep difficultly, and/or try to block it out. Then we progress to alcohol, medicine and even illegal drugs. Unfortunately, as one uses substances, which deaden the nervous system to reduce the perception of the pain, awareness of oneself and others are reduced in the process. Work, family and social activities are affected the negativity result makes the cycle of destructive mood, depression these events become closed-chain and traumatic.

In Our Everyday Experience
Experiences in 2000s are driving a car with one foot on the gas and the other on the brake. We experience stress at whatever time we initiate daily actions and hold it back at the same time. Our ever-obedient muscles try to obey both messages and work against each other. What great amount of vital energy is wasted and could be used in health and healing.

In the same way, we have our own unique muscular responses to the expression of emotions such as anger, sadness, fear and exhilaration. We use our muscles to block, control and restrain these strong feelings and our reaction to them. Even though we may be unaware of the amount of tension we store within, it puts the extra wear and tear on both mind and body over time.

Maintaining these patterns of chronic tension is like leaving the lights on all night-it takes energy; but once it's a habit, we no longer recognize it as such. What we do notice are the aches, pains, fatigue, headaches, digestive problems, PMS, or a host of other stress-related symptoms. These symptoms are important signals to be heeded, rather than ignored or bypassed. Accumulated stress and tension always diminish the amount of energy and vitality. We have to enjoy life, be creative and productive and strive for better things.

The antidote to stress is known as the relaxation response, which is triggered by the parasympathetic branch of the nervous system. This action sends messages to the body to relax slow down and take a deep breath: saying, in effect, it's time for rest and healing. However, we don't listen or pay attention.

There are a number of ways to promote effective responses, they include exercise, meditation, listening to calming music, guided visualization, biofeedback, and of course, the Love Touch.

The Love Touch Settings

The Love Touch should take place in a comfortable/safe environment, away from the many sources of the majority stressors and load noises. All of us need touch often. The latest research states that, "touch is as fundamental to the body as breathing air is essential to life."

As the Love Touch begins with the silky touch to stimulate the relaxation response, muscular tension is then released, circulation is increased and sensory receptors are activated. When this takes place the heart is beating slowly, and respirations are long and deep. Then the brain signals are chemically happy in joy, peace and loving emotions. Once you experience this piece go there once again and often.

Areas that have been "cut off" by accumulated stress can begin to feel normal once again. The Love Touch teaches us to tune into the body a signal that soothes us at the same time.

All of this greater body awareness will help us to more carefully monitor your own body's responses and needs. Then you can release tension before it becomes chronic and damaging as it builds up. Therefore, Living in a more relaxed and balanced body will enable you to handle the stresses in your life, and nothing can take you back to that state of well—being more quickly than The Love Touch and the knowledge you learn here.

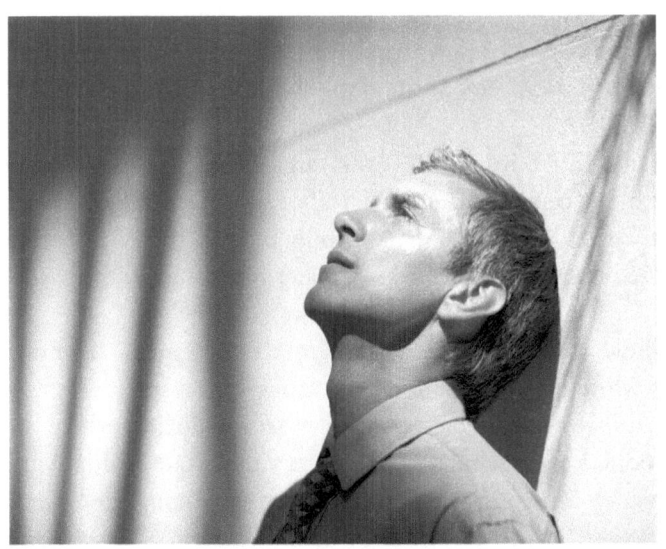

The Love Touch and Good Health

The Love Touch is a holistic therapy. It has major effect on both body and mind and gives positive effect to your spiritual being. The Love Touch will increase the circulation of blood and flow of lymph. The direct mechanical effect of rhythmically applied manual pressure and movement used in the Love Touch can dramatically increase the rate of blood flow. Furthermore, the stimulation of nerve receptors causes the blood vessels (by reflex action) to dilate, which also facilitates blood flow. This has a profound effect on one's health.

The key effects of the Love Touch.

Reduced muscle tension.
The Love Touch affects the muscles throughout the body.

The Love Touch will affect the muscle and connective tissues throughout the body. You learned methods will loosen contracted, shortened, hardened muscles. The methods will also stimulate weak, flaccid muscles. Chronic muscle tension reduces the circulation of the blood and movement of lymph, which is vital to balance.

The Love Touch improved blood circulation. The oxygen capacity of the blood can increase 10-15% after stimulation. By indirectly or directly stimulating nerves that supply internal organs, blood vessels of these organs dilate and allow greater blood supply to them.

The Love Touch causes better lymph movement. Lymph is a milky white fluid that drains impurities and wastes away from the tissue cells. A component of these wastes is toxins, which are the by-products of metabolism. So, it is a vital to our health. Muscular contraction has a pumping effect that moves lymph. The Love Touch and exercise help to move lymph. Lymph system other important is the T and B cells which fight virus and other forms of disease that are foreign to a human being.

The Love Touch will increase mobility and range of motion of joint:

The Love Touch provides a gentle stretching action to both the muscles and connective tissues that surround and support the muscles and many other parts of the body, which helps keep these tissues elastic.

The Love Touch will stimulate or soothed nervous system: The Love Touch helps balances the nervous system by soothing or stimulating it, depending on which effect is needed by the individual at the time of the processors.

The Love Touch enhances the skin condition by improving the function of the sebaceous and sweat glands, which keep the skin lubricated, clean, and cool. Youthfulness appears in the skin when it is stimulated and healthy.

The Love Touch will bring better digestion and intestinal function. The Love Touch increases the body's secretions and excretions. It increases the production of gastric juices, saliva, and urine.

There is also an increased excretion of nitrogen, inorganic phosphorus, and salt. As a result, the metabolic rate increases.

Kidney function will improve, and we will feel better all over.

The Love Touch will relieve acute and chronic pain.

The Love Touch can promote recovery from the fatigue and from minor aches and pains.

Other important benefits:
Beneficial effects on the internal organs and the immune system
Reduced swelling reduced stress General relaxation
Overall improvement in physical health and the quality of life.

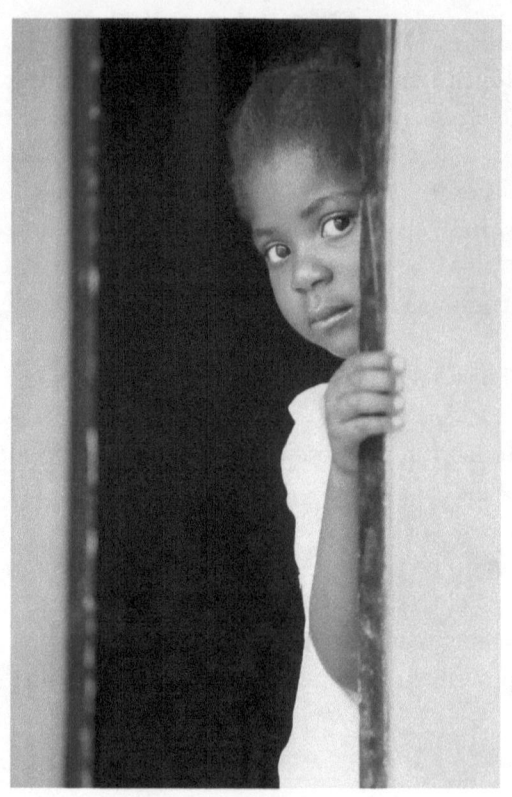

Historically

Research in massage therapy has been ongoing for more than 120 years. Here are some reported benefits of massage:

Students at the University of Medicine and Dentistry of New Jersey-New Jersey Medical Schools which were massaged before an exam showed a significant decrease in anxiety and respiratory rates. The students had the remarkable increase in white blood cells, and natural killer cell activity. Silence indicates a benefit to the immune system!

Preliminary results suggested cancer patients had less pain and anxiety after receiving the therapeutic massage at the James Cancer Hospital and Research Institute in Columbus, Ohio.

Women who had experienced the recent death of a child were less depressed after receiving the therapeutic massage, according to preliminary results of a study at the University of South Carolina.

Studies funded by the National Institutes of Health (NIH) have found massage beneficial in improving weight gain in HIV—exposed infants and facilitating recovery in patients who underwent abdominal surgery. At the University Of Miami School Of Medicine's Touch Research Institute, researchers have found that massage is helpful in decreasing blood pressure in people with hypertension, alleviating pain in migraine sufferers and improving alertness and performance in office workers.

An increasing number of research studies shows massage works!

The Love Touch reduces heart rate, lowers blood pressure, increases blood circulation and lymph flow, relaxes muscles, improves range of motion, and increases endorphins (enhancing medical treatment). Although therapeutic massage does not increase muscle strength, it can stimulate weak, inactive muscles and, thus, partially compensate for the lack of exercise and inactivity resulting from illness or injury. It also can hasten and lead to a more complete recovery from exercise or injury.

Research has verified that:
- Office workers love touch regularly were more alert, performed better and were less stressed than those who weren't love touch.
- Love touch decreased the effects of anxiety, tension, depression, pain, and itching in burn patients.

- Abdominal surgery patients recovered more quickly after love touch. Premature infants who were loved touched gained more weight and fared better than those who weren't.
- Autistic children showed less erratic behavior after love touch.

According to AMTA, love touch helps both physically and mentally. "Often time's people are stressed in our culture. Stress—related disorders make up between 80-and-90 percent of the ailments that bring people to family-practice physicians. What they require is someone to listen, someone to touch them, someone to care. That does not exist in modern medicine.

One of the complaints heard frequently is that physicians don't touch their patients any more. Touch just isn't there. Years ago massage was a big part of nursing and was used extensively in the cardiac units in German. There was care, so much touch, so much goodness conveyed through love touch. Now nurses, for the most part, are as busy as physicians. They're writing charts, dealing with insurance notes, they're doing procedures and often there is no room for love touches any more.

"I believe massage therapy is absolutely input to the healing process not only in the hospital environment, but because it relieves stress, it is obviously foundational in the healing process anytime and anywhere" (Joan Borysenko-Massage Journal Interview, Fall 1999).

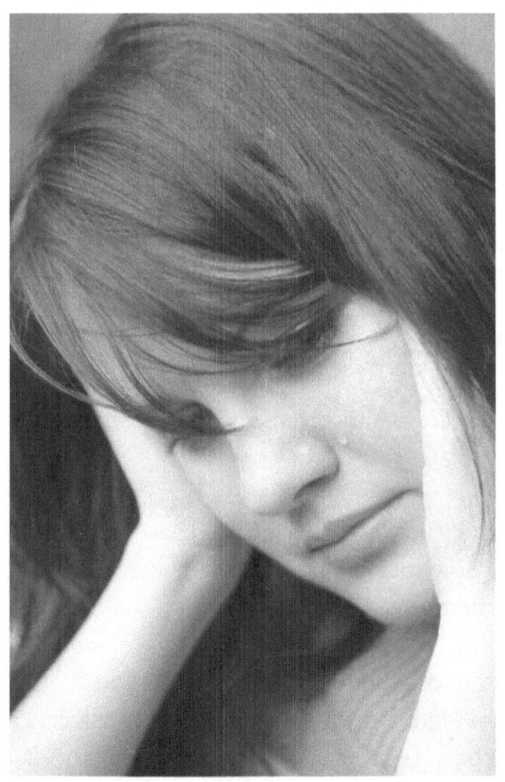

The Love Touch Importance in Healing and Balance

Come diseased, lonely, illness, and hurting to learn about The Love Touch. Learn that we are all deprived of Love Touch. Our loved ones need positive effects that The Love Touch will give to them, too. My concern for advancing simple healing, gives great comfort, peace of mind; which the healing actions were not insight, but were on its way? I hope and pray for the best to each who experiences The Love Touch. Each time I engage in the practice. I learn the importance of good technique and desire to get the most.

An excellent result occurred during these processes. I grow, in strength of intense of touch and increasing my knowledge of muscle response to touch. Mastering The Love Touch is no different from celebrated runner, bicyclers, swimmers or other illustrious athletic professions. Our experiences will achieve newness, because daily we change! All of us are healing! So, let's change positively.

It has taken me two years, to understand The Love Touch and its various touch strengths, many different techniques and new surprises that we'll discuss later.

Most surprising are positive changes for this will open your eyes and others to hope!

With a proper setting, you can grow and become very knowledgeable in relation to how touch is to us human's lives. Yes, touch is vital to balance. Furthermore, we strive for lasting wellness.

I have learned that the head is not the neck, and the feet are not the hands, and the right side of the body is really atypical from the left side, and the back is diverse as the front. Neck pain is nothing like back pain, and knee pain is not great toe pain, and tenuous elbow is different as gout in the knee. Each area has its needs for touch in its special way.

In addition, I have learned that muscles have a mind of their own when they are injured. What I'm saying is trauma muscle or spastic muscle does not a response every time you touch them. I appreciate and understand that the body system cycles itself. These areas worked on yesterday will reply with the same workout today, and it will change.

You might have to change technique and intensity or maybe even lighten up some. The body of the person that you work on will help dictate the most comfortable technique and intensity on each session. You will learn as you experience this human need for touch changes, and that will come after you learn about the body's cycling and its need to work towards balance.

Americans are full of anger and stress! Anger that lives within people, inside their very being, and exhibit itself in life as serious problems; most often as diseases/cancers. Actually, these uptight and irritated people have experienced hurts, traumas in their life and need The Love touch. In reality, many of these people are our family members, co-workers; on the highway . . . road rage and even you're daily shopping experiences.

American Advertises Companies are promoting sex too young and old Americans. Sex is under the cover of clothes, make-up, music, stores, sit-com, magazines, tabloids, computer and other newsprint's. Chat rooms, negative web sites and text messages on add to the stress. Young Americans have never experienced pondering or day dream. There are priceless monuments combat stress and weariness. Buying into the sex/electronic life-style is not wholesome, because the healthy body needs balance. Unbalanced people do not sleep well. Sleep is important to healing and balance. The Love Touch can help reverse the unhappy stresses while helping to brake the cycles of stress. Once your body becomes discerning; healing is in the wings! Losing stressful emotion will add to your strengths. Ever time your thoughts get away from stress. This is precious monument work toward healing, because the body wants to be whole! Some people call it being centered or balanced.

Touch is essential to us ALL! Not all of us Americans believe that touch is crucial to a balance life! Even so, the Love Touch gives you understanding in words and touch therapy experiences. Research has shown us that all of us have needs! If you were at a general meeting and ask how many people have aches and pains from back pain, knee pain, ankle pain, foot pain, finger pain, hand pain, arm pain, shoulder pain, neck pain, headaches . . . a good 80% of the meeting people would experience basic daily pains and aches. I hope that you get the picture; that we all could have a positive experience with the simple touch. A worker cannot work at their most excellent when they chronically experience discomfort or in continuous pain.

Research has shown us that we think an even day on three to four important subjects. We start each day with 12 or more thoughts or subjects while waking up except we are not intelligent enough to think satisfactory on more than two subjects most of the day. So when we experience trauma, strains/stress and pains, it captures a lot of our attention. The Love Touch can brake these vicious cycles! Pains continue every minute and hours of the day, every day, every week and month and the pain has a mine of its own for life is not good. Examples are back pain/injuries know about sitting uncomfortable, because there is no easy chair; there are no relaxed sleeping positions; even the floor does not sleep well; these people know about no relief from pain by using prescription medicines and/or surgeries.

Most of the time injuries give pains from a specific area. However, experience has shown me that the pain area may not be the trigger point. It often means that something else is out of aliment or dysfunctional. The Human body works as a unit. When there is an illness in the body the whole body knows it and tries' to compensate. One therapist states it this way: "many times physicians would send an order to work on the knee and the knee was not the source of injury" "I have to examine and find the source" and "then the knee heels!"

When we get surgery, it is trauma! When we fall down that is trauma. When we feel hurt it is trauma, too. When we take many pills, it is not health it is trauma! When we eat too much this is trauma. Trauma comes in various shapes, sizes and habits; however, they all affect us differently. Therefore, Medicines should place on the scales of justice! There you can see the truth about medicines; they have helpful qualities; and yet side effects are many times worse than the overall helping aspect of the medicine. Sometimes helpful portions far out perform the side effect. Only the patient knows! I have a very sensitive body, and I do not like the metallic taste I have with medication. Aspirin works better for me then hard narcotics. Pain medicine will not kill the pain of inflammation! Medicine only mast the pain not removed it. Fibromyalgia and other contact tissue diseases live with enormous joint and body discomforts daily. Many drugs do not work on contact tissue disease. That is why The Love Touch is so important here.

Some of these auto-immune diseases experience nerve blocks. Nerve blocks are very painful and often unsuccessful. Losing feeling in areas that use to have pain is not success!

Infrequently pain or disease gives us the initial source of dysfunction or brakes down area within the connective tissue or organ. We must try to find the one or two trigger points. Trigger points are not necessary memory cells. However, both cell types need to recognize forester healing. These trigger points when affected at the right time, and space give grand changes in our fight for wellness.

Insight-fullness will teach us that one-day something good will happen and I will change. Sometimes these changes take week, months and even years; however, leaving each day in hope gives a vision that points the way to balance. That is the day we work towards wholeness.

I have learned that trigger points will come alive, once they are attention too. It's not that simple you will have to work to find it. I believe that the body wants to be whole. I believe that the body wants to help it make you healthy. DNA has written the code. Inflammation, trauma, or injury alters the skeletal systems! These changes can be acute, chronic or result from an episode that changes the structure to make them abnormal. Now pain and spasms last and they affect your sleep and bowel habits; we have long, and life is hard with general bad days. Your energy is not there, because depression sits in. Remember let's work with DNA, who is still in control! Let's work to find the trigger points. With the DNA, found trigger points we work toward health and balance.

Modern Medicine has incorporated emotions and its affection on healing. Visualizing a good result and believe that their treatment is given by the distinguished medical team. Wound healing shows the less nerve-racking people heal 7-10 days faster than those under continues stress. These examples have added to my belief that we all have too much chatter in our brains. Calm peaceful minds heal quicker. Add cellular phones/electronics trouble activity continued. We all need to brake the stressful cycles!

The Love Touch can be special touch will relax the body, respirations decrease, and then you notice you are not thinking at 278 miles an hour. You notice that your body is quite . . . body wanted to be quiet! The body can find its way home! Relax!

Unfortunately, every day you get stress while spasms cycles and intensity changes. Intensity changes in injury because lactic acid is produced in the copy's amount from sick muscles. Convulsive muscles cause toxic waste as a result of pain; aching-intense spastic pain. Particularized personality pains are subjective to personality; however, pain can be scaled by intelligent guest work as a physician. Patience knows their pain and how it felt!

Epsom salt bath can help remove lactic acid. It far inferred wearable can remove lactic acid from skeletal muscle quickly. If these modalities are will help in your healing, then you will be changed. Our goal is to increase full range of motion to the injured area. Unhealthy bodies need increase blood circulation to add to healing quotient.

Always, the body knows what is right; however most of us do not pay attention, because we want to eat, think and do what we want. While practicing emergency medicine, I noted patience's disease that slowly took the life out of them. Claudicating from disease of the arteries of the lower leg; skeletal muscle "cry" like the heart does when it is starving of oxygen, because of the lack of health blood supplies.

These diabetic patience's have pain on walking. Walking is critical to good health. One 80's year-old men has a resting pulse of 59/ minuet. He walks everyday and takes no medicine. Walking to the mail box becomes difficult. When these patience's are treated and vascular circulation improves life.

When a health change comes sometime they change dreadful habits that cause the problem. Those who do not change distressing habits will not become balanced.

The Head is the most valuable structures of the human body. These rounds house the brain and on top the hair! The brains in general autonomic it thinks and reacts while orchestrating controls our bones, connects with the nerves, vascular systems and lymphatic.

The Head sits upon the top of our human body structure. Unfortunately, stress settles at the nape or base of the neck/head and at the bottom of our feet. Hands and finger cramp up, shoulders get tight. Over time, we wear a tired head/neck muscle, and arthritis comes.

The feet, knees, and hip get tired and hurt. Now we are sick. Then we get headaches, neck pain, hip pain, knee pain and feet ache. Love Touch the head and neck and the body relaxes, and intense pains wane. It is important to know that by decreasing the severity of pain allows the additional range of motion-movements, healing sleep, and more energetic days. This is what I want for each person that hurts and live with pain to have some relief! Now is the time to embrace good thoughts of balance.

Emotions live with us! Well-behaved emotions are important to healthiness! You are your emotion! Nevertheless, you have choices!

Different choices on the new emotions unlike the ones you live with now. Those present emotions will drive you out of your normal health state and keep you stress and full of disease. When I meet people who have the auto-immune disease like lupus or other connect tissue disease. Ask them if they have been divorced, death in the family, lost a job, had to move and there are many more stresses? Divorce causes stress in people who continually learn to live with it! Why not let hurt, anger, and pain go? Learn how important right thoughts are too good emotions and health.

Who would want a person that caused you pain . . . to run your life/our emotions? Some people are like a duck. Ducks allow water (stress) roll down their downy feathers fast! The Love Touch will allow the body's emotion to relax sooner than later and work toward home . . . balance!

As you participate in The Love Touch, you will be alive touched physically, emotionally, and spiritually. When you care about someone, have understood trust come into play! Commanding result will come with trust, because you will touch areas that could not be without trust. True trust comes from God. God loved us and our love should be like Jesus Love, so we can trust Him! Trust promotes brotherly love. Love shared that passes all understanding/ unconditional enormous results is inevitable.

Conversation and dialog will play an important part in The Love Touch. Dialogue that dealt with touch and feeling! "How does this feel"? Linger for the spoken response, and then adjust if necessary. You want to be a barometer to know how you touch affects your family member or partner. We are working together for the best! Respectable communications can only add to the quality of The Love Touch. We want the remarkable result every session of The Love Touch.

Some days you will be unintentional not within the "Ball Park" of trust, caring, and understand. However, one or two of you will work forward and that day may be the impressive day of The Love Touch. Accordingly, the magic of believing will show something good will comes out of all experiences in The Love Touch.

Those who take The Love Touch to heart will grow in strength and character, and then become a faithful and trusting a person in time! Greater true friend ship will come with these experiences and commitments. We all need each other to heal! Allow healing plus hope to work with the touch to spread it all over. Yes, spread to others that are destitute of touch.

All human bodies cry for touch! Please, touch me tenderly soft and often! Touch me and make me whole! Touch me and we will grow old together! Love me with the touch and we will be alive! So often loneliness masses the need for touch, because a hurt feels are frequently not known the source from which it comes.

You who are inexperienced at message, physical therapy, have your hairs worked on or any type of body touch; you will have a remarkable experience because you want to be better or work towards balance. The novice touch person can have a great experiencing touch and sharing with others. They will help him become more loving, kind and at the end of the day work to balance. Anyone can have good experience with The Love Touch. Anyone who cares about others and knows the service is an honorable duty.

Why should we stay the same? Why should we stay sick and unbalanced? Anyone who has reached a level of health or performances will tell you that life is never stagnated! Life is daily cyclic with active emotion and ever changing! Those who languish will rust out, burn-out, and become a couch potato! Those who want a balance and first-class level of health attitude will likely work for a good result daily! The Love Touch people will work for high-quality! Intelligent people wants balance, happiness and wholeness! Wholeness is an attainable goal! Those who go there have daily peaceful lives! I want to be on the winning side, don't you? Let's start today on your way to balance!

Many patients have you been told that you must live with your illness/diseases, take our pills and exist on for the rest of your time! Alternatively, you are getting old! Those who buy into the disease, pills and live with symptoms will have them until they decide to look for other treatment, therapies and cures. I want to teach you to say, "My doctor says that I have diabetics or some other disease." However, I am working to wellness or balance. Yes, there is something that will help your illness. Little changes can bring large changes in time! Believe this and you won't be sorry!

Because Americans have the finest health system, yet we have more diseases and stress than other countries. Most Americans are unhappy, depressed, and live with many stressful issues. They live each day sad and depressed! Sadness and depression are not what they are cracked up to be! I have learned that being fantastic each day gives me vital energy and hope. Hope and energy for what I cannot see. I believe that my attitude is important; then I do my part help the DNA in my body to work. In returns, the bodies work to the best that it can do! No one knows why some heal, and others do not. I believe that positive attitude and Hope make the possible play in the mine to my happy child inside. If your child in the side is sad, hurt, anger, depressed, fearful, shame . . . you need touch for it will help you. Furthermore, touch will make you happy and peaceful like a child on the inside. It is important to good health. Happy Children have hope. We, adults need Hope! Add laughter to you day 300 times and this will give you joy.

One of the biggest secrets of achievement is in the journey. You won't be dissatisfied if you relax let it be happy! Most achievements are hard-work. However, there is notable blessing in helping others. Smell the rose along your path! Each step every day will take you there . . . balance . . . good sleep . . . and much more.

Let's work together in love and grow in trust then share new insights and adjustment in are experience of The Love Touch. Some may believe that group sessions are critical. However, what is vital are remarkable insights experienced in proper sessions?

We want to have the benefit of these high-quality experiences because The Love Touch is for our own excellent! The more Americas that are touched the happier we will be! Children who are starving for touch . . . one touch and twice touched will help the anger and lonesomeness inside

Do you want a positive attitude? For it is positive attitude aids in healing. Positive attitude becomes a requirement to those who want to be balanced. This means emotions of spiritual, physical, attitude are affected positively. Can this happen all at once? No! One day at a time in the spirit of love-positive attitude can be obtained. Many people attempt to work on one aspect of their life and then another part; they don't understand why the body. Its parts are not getting where you want them to go. So go in confidence! Work in optimistic! Think in encouraging! Live in affirmative! Positive thought will affect the DNA and the Brain. Naturally, two parts of the body will work together for good results will occur . . . yes! Believe it to achieve it! See the unsurpassed! Expect the Finest! Be the best!

Strength comes with good Love Touch experiences. First-hand experience with another human being who in turn want the same results; that is great! So get started looking for, good experiences, essential energy, and happier days to come soon! The future is tomorrow or even minutes henceforth. Come let me take you there. This is The Love Touch!

I started The Love Touch by running my finger through my girl friend's blond hair. The fingers give a lift to the hair which gives a good sensation to the scalps and delightful emotion of care. I watched her face become peaceful, respirations lessen, and relaxation comes over her in minutes at each session. This first Love Touch experiences surprised me! The more I, message her neck, scalps, and hair remarkable relief of tension and stress, and she got better sleep. Now when I touch her scalp and neck, peaceful sessions occur, because she was in a relax state, with proper breathing and a less stressful state. Each Love Touch experience became different, because my fingers have grown in strength.

Muscle strength gave the increase finger pattern that because more change in tightness in the scalp and neck. Many sessions surprise me over and over, because The Love Touch becomes alive to me, and I want an excellent result . . . that came with time. Additionally skillful touch intensity and rhythms grow and vary nobility teaching the importance of good technique. New and authoritative experiences are important in your Love Touch experience! When you reach these level's surprises and change you will have arrived at higher levels this will astonish you!

Weeks later you will notice a physical change in your stamina, in your muscle strength and tone. Your partners will fill the difference and appreciate your level of new achievement. A result will be elevation and your trust and understand to grow. Now with your new improved positive attitude your Love Touch experiences will give them better sleep, most important energy and much improved balanced days. Many Americans never experience the great level of the human spirit that comes ultimately from God! God is Love! All positive healing comes from God. Many Christians who lack the Love Touch will reach new heights when they incorporate it into their families.

All these positive changes excite me that am why I spend so much of my life in the service to elevate people's awareness and importance of The Love Touch!

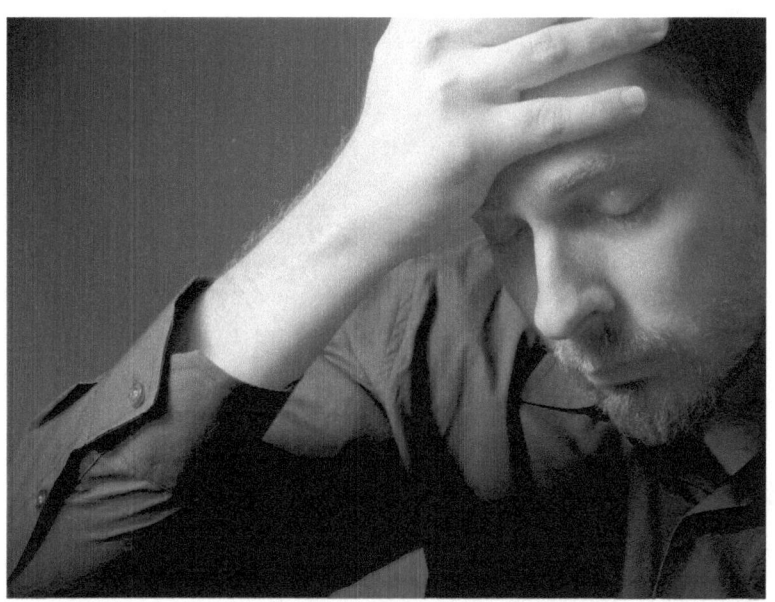

Personal Awareness!

Why do we buy into that which we cannot understand or find purpose in? Dark color soda/pops, diet soda/ pop, and they help demineralization bone and make us fat. Dark sodas/pops have the ph same as Meramec acid ph of 1.5 very acidic. Dark sodas/pops affected the kidneys by stressing the epithelial cells. Epithelial cell are important for healthy kidneys. Additionally, those who drink dark sodas/pops cause inflamed Urinary tract. Young women who drink dark sodas/ pops have chronically abnormal UTI; which create concern by Gynecological doctors who now think kidney failure. Kidney failure diagnoses are by kidney biopsy. Biopsy is not a benign procedure.

Every time, you drink dark sodas/pops you should drink 30 glasses of water to clear each 12 oz dark sodas/pops from you toxic body.

So let's stop the dark sodas/pops and returns to a normal kidney by drinking water. Many diseases are caused by outside toxins . . .

remove these damaging chemical substances and your health will change for the better.

The Love Touch people will notice changes in muscle strengths in short time if you 're working experience are two or more times per week. This should not surprise you if you have ever worked out before. Most men do not take much effect to increase muscle tone; women muscle tone just a little slow, however, they will change in good time. Once you experience change rhythm will change too. Soon, you will include rhythmus of life and will support the immune system. Rhythms of life are soft and else going and nothing like hard, loud speedy stress. Unaware that The Love Touch is taken stresses to redden body on the way to balance. Stress and worry have destroyed the human spirit, and so many live are now depression and loneliness. Divorced people, widows, and many stressed single people have heart attaches.

Couples and families become good friends have good times together, long to please each other, and grow in trust and love. These people have Love Touch in their lives. Often, I witness Joe, at my church. Joe continually touches the neck of his young children while sitting in the pews at church. They are a happy and agreeable balanced family. Children are enjoyable and pleasing pleasant to talk to.

Look at your hands! Understand how important they can be for serving a friend or love one! Imagine that you have energy that keeps you alive; however, this mighty energy . . . far infrared is the warmth in your hands! This dominant far-infrared wave length comes from the Sun. The oscilloscope, visualizes energy wave length on a color screen. Colors range from green with yellows and reds and hot white! If you place your hands on the walls and then remove them; the screen will show reds and yellows patterns on the wall. Your energy will transfer it to the wall. Well, we can do the same thing to people we touch?

Just, an image that your friend or the person you what to help is not looking well today.

Their skin is pale and wasted! Not enough sleep, lots of coffee/ cigarettes; or besides junk-food; or too much alcohol and working without understanding! Now, too many sports and porno; this is sad! You do not know what thoughts, emotional stress and/or sicknesses are consuming their present mood! They want to be alone! This is heartbreaking because mopping and warring around only makes the situation worse. Talking will not move the chronic cycling of involuntary muscle; however, a loving touch can move mountains! I remember the rubbing of my chest and feet with Vicks when I had a cold as a child! Well! I was much better in the morning; because I believe what my dad did for me was making it easier for me heal quickly. Discomforts of illness over power healing hands with far infrared! Good energy always helps displacement of bad energy!

Every time, I think about how dad loved us, while care about our needs! I get happy, warm, and peaceful. Healing feeling and thought help healed us! Often, I see these patterns of stress in my family; I place my hand around the back of the neck and leave it there for several seconds. Anticipation as well as patience is commanding tools in The Love Touch! You will learn how authoritative they are as you grow in the Love Touch. Start with soft hand at the base of the neck noticed the tightness of muscle and softness of connective tissue. Usually, the strapped muscles run from the basic of the skull to the c-spine and thoracic spine. The neck and head are motivated by these muscles. Muscles need a lot of touch and through this work, you will see good results. Then you will understand why!

Music is a notable tool. Music can touch the soul by giving relaxing moods. It helps drive away the uncontrollable emotions that we have had since 7 years old. Yes, love touch gives needed optimistic accents! Affirmative tone of voice or instrument in music moves at paces and rhythm that will help move stressed muscles and stressed emotions.

Make possible your Love Touch muscle to work diligently for change. Changes that will strengthen you and cause a good result in our positive love touch experience. The Love Touch never feels because it can help change the person in most important need. Music with drums also adds to the healthy mix for optimal success. I personally like to Love Touch with mood music, which allow our fingers to work with the beat of the drums or accents of the solo. This is the rhythmus of the universe. Muscles like these movements as well as the person working these actions.

Thank goodness that we can glean from important body signs that show us the way as a result of giving us the hidden road map. If the signs are present during the love touch, they maybe apply now or to next The Love Touch action. What are some of these important signs? Notice the skin color and texture; count the respirations, because when you start the Love Touch skin than respirations will change as well as the color of the skin. Supplementary body change will present to person's conciseness. When the receptions have reached a satisfied level then trust and relaxation follow. Levels of rest will come during the sessions. These levels of relief make the reception feel youthful and alive. Still other sign may be cracking, popping, along with other new-found sounds. I have notice at the list seven difference sounds in my healing body. So pay attention and you will learn to teach others the important sign, too.

Several times over the last year I discovered that your greatest rhythms and intensity movement does not appear right (for help that diseased muscle) over the spastic muscles. So I changed gears and use your palm or just your fingers. Now the muscle gives. It doesn't always work that way. You might have to change movement again until the muscles except the challenge. There are great areas of the body that work well with other parts of the love touch person. Rolfer's use their elbows; just think how authoritative the elbow is! And it works well!

Fingers are exiting because they have special touch technique. Fingers are sensitive, and will work individually over areas of the back. Afterward use a spider works and grab an area like a ball except the loser and hold gently. Play muscles like a piano! I will validate!

What would you like to say after the first Love Touch experience? It appears as if I beyond doubt am living for the first time. Understanding, that your wonderful body is alive! You lost the past in addition to future all at the same time! You finely have been live in the moment of time. Dedicated people sent many years meditating, in quiet time, and pray to get toward balance and the LOVE TOUCH can take you there! Understanding changes, because Love Touch works together so each partner gets good results.

Once you have mastered these straightforward tools of life it will be better for you and your Love Touch partner on the road to good health. Now you're can understand Mother Theresa, who love the untouchable in her country and make many of the health and whole.

Important History!

In 1785, C. E. Savary, the Frenchman after experiencing massage in Egypt so wisely stated: There is a lively feeling of existence, which radiates to the extremities of the body, be aware of the wholeness that is given over to the delightful sensations; the takes cognizance of these, and enjoys the agreeable thoughts; the imagination wanders over the universe which it adorns, sees smiling pictures, the image of happiness.

Love Touch will give you experience that money cannot buy!

Today's Life!

Most Americans have lots of chatter in their busy brains; and are always thinking about something or some person or some situation or issue. We need quiet times, to break the traumatic emotions that drive us in the wrong direction, making us and are unhealthy. One of the prominent new mean noted that people in 2006 do not day dream anymore; this is the price of electronics, phones, tech-messages, eating poorly and living in stress! Day dreaming is an authoritative tool in helping develop positive people who live good lives. Day dreaming is an important element to combine with the Love Touch in working toward balance.

Today is the new day! What will you do with it? Will you play in the past and think how much it hurts or cries because no one else is feeling what you feel? What an illustrious pity party that makes you worst and depressed. It's about time that these experiences get old. Stop giving your life to trauma, illness, old time, lost friends, lost loved one, bad experience, and not understand that you are only in control of your next decision. Yes, you have the right to choose not to believe that issues in life are for real. That events or issue in your life does not affect your physical body. From the beginning of The Love Touch, I have proven to you how important touch, is to the Human body.

Every day Researchers, Watch Groups and the FDA tell how awful our processed foods are. Grain's vitamins are wasted during processes and then replaced with vitamin A & D. Whole grain maintains the true vitamin and nutrition that we need to be in good health. Whole grains, fruits and vegetables make the healthiest diet. Some have called the health diet . . . God's diet compares to the unhealthy nutritional lacking, fatty, wasted out American Diet. Health Diets are important to sustaining good life. Simple, color, clean foods are the paramount diet to promote and accelerate your balance adventure. Just think and believe that balance is possible! It's celebrated that your adventure will be your own!

Research shows that we are hardwired to need touch in our early developmental stages (Field, 1995). The Industrial Revolution caused related changes in child-rearing practices and has altered illustrious Westerns care for and connected with these babies.

Fears of mothers in the 80s began sitting in the back seat through their 1-5-year old children. Then mothers allowed the very young children to sleep in their beds. These women over protected the child, causing these children to have impressive fears. This traumatism their everyday lives. Children need to know that you are there. Nevertheless, they need time alone to grow, experience life and mature as they, adventure through their new lives. Several women on Oprah Show in April, 2006, talked about their stress in dealing with their young ones. They state that their children never get to see their mother happy, because we are too busy doing.

Yes, happiness has been taken over by business and achieving daily goals and not doing simple possessions like touch, understanding, and communications at the right time. The best to do is lift your spirit and the ones around you. Take time to smell the roses. Choose values in life that support health family and individual happiness.

Twenty-four-hour Televisions and Computers are baby-sitting the very young. Researchers know that we are what we see and embrace. Eighty percent of what we do in our lives is come from what we see and experience not what we know. Apple's seeds do not grow oranges. However, often we do not know or believe the truths about our behavior. We only see what we want to see. Vast example of eating behavior was first noted in those whom eat like a bird. Those

65-pound ladies with fasting blood sugars of 45 points [normal 110] looked unhealthy only saw their way of life perfect. One research took a photo of one lady. The first time she saw here a photo, "That is not me!" It took six months of repeat photo to get the lady to realize that her condition was not normal. There are millions of the stories with like above-mentioned patterns of dis-functionless. It is healthy to have friend or family that is honest with their feeling and then. The Love Touch helps by allowing stress and negative about energy be vented over time.

Good health habits are essential to all of us! We are all human and come from America's melting pot or other countries. We all have the basic same needs loved, hungry, enough sleep, in good physical shape, and socially accepted by your workers, family and friends. People have no time for exercise or no time to cook something healthy. People are still stressed by experience and have lots of issues with families and others. Come make good for your health choices, and we will have success!

The Importance of Good Music

Music is important for good life, because it allowed us to escape into your imaginative mind; there is healing here. Healing because it breaks the stress filled days with moments of peace and tranquility. Find the music that gives you fundamental energy in vision. Not the hot music that makes you work hard, dance and move your body. We are not looking for exercise, but music that stimulate nurturing and wholeness.

Lyrical instrument plays a rhythmic music that relaxes our busy minds. Now, let's experience The Love Touch while these peaceful poetic songs play.

Music will allow its rhythmus ways to help your essential hand and finger movement. Watch the Love Touch person and increase your knowledge of positive outside stimulus ability's aide in healing. Classical music works will. However, you find many other types and or style of music that will work well too. Music without words wills assistant (both) the receiver and the touch person in working in concert.

They are outstanding stories about patients with coma for weeks. Someone comes to the bed side and plays heart description melodies that cause the patient's heart rate strengthen, skin pinks-up, and the eyes brighten. Music has the encouraging power! We need helpful power with The Love Touch. Synergism state that two parts (powerful music & The Love Touch) result will be greater than anticipated.

Image the fantastic sounds of Classical music: Maestro will you heal with your hands you will touch with care the skin of other, who needs the healing touch! You touch with your fine fingers and walk across the surface of the back of the head. You will notice that the skull is not smooth! Are their muscles on the scalps that are bumpy? These bumpy are areas causing elevated tension! Then you need circular finger movement to help release tension caused by stress. Heads and necks hold a lot of tension. Relieve the tension on the skull and positive reaction will occur over the whole body.

Learn to use accessible balance within the hand and finger!

How can I make such statements that are of outstanding results? I am a medical scientist, who continually looks for healing answers. Albert Einstein and other celebrated scientists believe that "the answer is in the question." Ask first-class questions than good-quality answers will come; not always at once but keep looking and believe then you won't be real disappointed. Harmonious hand and finger movements playing like the piano, individual transfer to the reception's body a positive technique.

About one and half years ago, I started the love touch. It started with the running my fingers through my best friend's blond hair. This technique made her scalp and hair alive. I also noticed that this middle age thin shapely lady cares her head down. The shoulder sloped, and the overall spine resembling one, who worked with their hands for years. When I questioned her about her diagnosis carpel tendentious, she gives the additional history of a cut left thumb, fracture nasal bones, vertigo, jaw cracking, left hand and upper extremities fall asleep at will, lower back ache, left hip pain, groin pain and fibromyalgia.

On the exam, I noticed that muscle on the right shoulder was greater than the left. Shoulders are forward, and the head is not sitting high on the shoulders. This look caused by trauma from many years of standing working with her hands; (1st) cutting hair for years and

(2nd) working in a metal factory on a machine. When people work around machinery the human body takes on the pessimistic energy exposed to them. This harmful energy removes critical energy from the human and causes crucial injury to their muscles, spirit, and emotions. People who work years in these situations lose normal body structure, which makes them vulnerable to diseases.

Often, I Love Touch her scalp. First, there were tender connective tissue and muscle sheets areas where the neck and head anatomically work together at the suture lines. Most importantly noted at this time was the then top of the scalp where little more tender than the rest of the scalp. These tender areas need soft Love Touch until the scalp is ready to change. With each meeting area of tendentious that changed new ones appear. I believe that these continually changes are layers of disease or pain coming off. Most disease does not change all at once them, stair step backwards from the initial onset of pain or illness.

When I am applying touch to the neck and scalp stress is released! I got huge results. Results included the lady having greater sleep, hair growing faster, and left arm did not fall asleep as often. When I touch the c-spine and thoracic spine area; I work with both hands noticing the posterior shoulder, neck muscles, and notice tender spots. I used my finger with good results. Straightaway, I used fingers like a type writer faster, then slowly. Muscles have a mind of their own. Muscle's change over time by stress and injury causes altered functional muscle. However, noted differential muscle purposes. I believe that the body wants to be balance and health. It will work towards balance if, we do the right features. Good health habits and style and eating colors will help the body heal.

Muscles, tendons, bones have immense pain or discomfort, when they are injured. Sprain ankle will cause your body to shift or adjust to the traumatic changes. These changes cause more energy, because when our bodies are working will, it is easy! When trauma comes our attention is misplaced and not concerned about the rest of the body!

Edema causes engorgement body connective tissue. It takes three weeks for these traumas to heal. However, it is not health to maintain the residual swelling. Swelling or spasms cause the tendon, muscles and bones to function under pressure. Additionally, Lactic acid builds from chronic spasms; there toxins cause achy pain. Pain medicine will not remove these unnerving aching pains. Pains get worse at night!

Ida Rolf an engineer from MIT believed that our spine change overtime because of gravity and many traumas during our life. Eventually, the Spinal changes causing arthritis c-spine, thoracic-spine, and lumbar spine and our organs become out of balance. When this happens, life is hard, and continuous stress only adds to this imbalance.

It is important to understand that the body wants to be healthy. When you start touching the body, you will understand that muscles need to be lead to wellness. The body is in rebellion when sick or diseased! The body has learned to live unbalance; it takes time and effects to move back to balance. Surprise and attack, I call it! This means soft methodical movement then quick almost abrasive movement. These techniques will teach you a variety. We will learn more about these techniques later. To be shown!

Why Are Feet Important?

Feet

Feet are important! The body is a huge unit of Billion of cells that function as One Human body. You can see on the above Feet Reflexology Chart. It is astonishing that the feet will give good results that affect others parts or sites of the body. Feet may be the only part of the body that will give you the workable result this day. Changing from the scalp-c-spine to the feet or from the feet to the lumbar spine gives the variety to cause quick healing.

However, the walk is not straight. You will have to learn how to attack the muscles.

That means functioning at optima. You will in due course learn when and where to attack each muscle group.

Feet

My life: medicine training, respiratory care experience, denier (autopsies) skills, author books, public speaker preventive health and inventor non-invasive medical device. Who as a child first believed in hope, care, kindness, and wellness and balanced. Medicine educators believe that mathematics scores on the med cat are important to diagnosis. Good Physicians are scientists who are always looking for new understanding of illness/disease processes. Appreciative thought of disease and balance there is but the little difference because both come from cause and effect. What will I do today to work toward a health life-style? What can I remove from my bad habits, which will move me in the directions of balance? Inch by inch anything a cinch!

Several days ago the lady had celebrated changes in her scalp. When this occurred muscled in the c-spine, thoracic spine started to (change) give and move. Muscle that was very tender to touch now became supple. Untimely nice lady's head has come up and shoulder back, and she glides in her gate. While working on lady's scalp, I started noticing that her skin on her face and hands engorged. Her blood vessels became erythematosus with a new youthful look. This look continues while I love touch and spread to the hands and rest on the total body. This lowers hydrocystine, adrenaline and others stress hormones. Oh, how we want to prevent diseases and chronic illness.

Let's look at several different methods of the Love Touch. First, we learn to touch with understanding and notice our bodies and the need for touch. Then we learn that different areas of the body need touch together with other areas and/or even by itself. We will learn when multiple groups well help changes that in synergism give a greater result. Solitary area touch methods are rare. Only time will dictate distinct touch work areas. These are newly traumatized area and need our attention now.

Touch is vitally important growth and development of good healthy bodies: the underlying mechanisms for the effects of touch are unknown, positive effects have been noted for many growths, development and health phenomena as the following few examples will show.

Children with autism are described as being extremely sensitive and averse to touch. However, they appear to accept massage, perhaps because it is predictable. In one study on preschool children with autism, their disruptive behavior in the classroom decreased. Their ability to relate to their teachers increased after a 10-day period of massage. In a second study, parents massaged their autistic children every night. The children experienced the same benefits as in the first study, but their sleep also improved [7]. Massage could well be a basic way to reach out to these children who appear to reject adult attention and affections.

Massage can also help alertness. In a job-stress study, the staff and faculty of a medical school were massaged for 15 minutes a day for a month, during their lunch breaks. We recorded their EEG patterns before, during and after the massage session. Their alpha and beta wave levels decreased, while the theta increased, supporting the feeling of heightened awareness reported by the subjects. We also tested their performance on math computations. After the massage, they took significantly less time to do the tasks, and their accuracy increased [8]. Perhaps massage breaks should become as institutional as coffee breaks!

Massage therapy has noted a reduce pain in various pain syndromes. Children with juvenile rheumatoid arthritis experience chronic pain because their anti-inflammatory medication is often on partially effective, and they cannot be prescribed narcotics, because of the risk of addiction. A 1-month studied parent who gave daily massages to their rheumatoid arthritis children. They noted positive effects: anxiety and stress levels decreased, as did the pain. There are explanations for the reduced pain.

The pressure nerves stimulated by the massage may send their message faster to the brain than the pain receptors, thus closing a 'gate' and preventing the reception of the pain message. Another possibility is increased production of serotonin, which has both antidepressant and anti-pain properties.

In addition, massage therapy has noted a decrease in symptoms in immune disorders such as asthma, diabetes and dermatitis and to enhance immune function, most particularly the production of natural killer cells that ward off cancer and viral cells [1].

Another study noted that moderate-pressure touch is necessary for these effects to occur. Moderate-pressure touch stimulates pressure receptors which in turn stimulate the vagal (one of the 12 cranial nerves) and increase vagal activity. This leads to a slowed heart rate and lower blood pressure, and the general behavioral effect is a relaxed, more attentive state. Other touch effects noted to include a reduction in stress hormones (Cortisol is a primary example), which could improve immune function, since Cortisol normally kills natural killer cells. We also see an increase in activating neurotransmitters, including serotonin and dopamine, and the alterations in EEG patterns which, I have already mentioned.

Is there any dough that touch is important to each, I? Therefore, take these thought and allow them to move you forward in the goodness of life. Continually working for the good of ourselves and others, because we are not alone and we all need each other. Daily promote health, happiness and peace of mind to all. Peace is happy, while touching in love.

Well-behaved health habits are important to overall health balance. If you what to learn more about favorable health habits "Eating to Win" can help you and your family inhabit healthy balanced lives. The best of health to you and all who learn and use these health tips along with The Love Touch.

We are all children and we need mentoring, helping hands, understanding and The Love Touch. Sharing these new-found insights result in powerful feeling when another hurting person finds relief. A smile can be the sparkles that get hope started. So, do it again and one more time! Make a believer out of others. Allow the smiles and sparkle to unite others to this noble cause!

Now that you have read The Love Touch are convinced that the Central Nerves (Brain) can be moved by the largest organ in the human body? Moreover, by applying simple daily Love Touch really works? By now, you are thinking out of the box. Will you raise a flag for victory over stress, depression and diseases?

Will you place your thoughts in the wastebasket of your cluttered mine? Step from the stage of mediocrities, then jump for joy that you are a Love Touch Stage that continually works in Hope. A Human Being is a person who has the insights of Life. We are. even so, but different and we all need The Love Touch. The Love Touch stage is not perfect but has what we all need. Could you ask for more? The Love Touch satisfies a down-to-earth need; therefore, it can be given freely to all. This includes the Stressed and Depressed Americans!

Your rewards for becoming a Love Touch person are much greater than anyone can predict, because the joy of simulating hope in others is very satisfying. You sleep better, food will taste enhanced, your attitude will become positive, and your horn of plenty will be filled. Yes, thinking out of the box can be rewarding. Remember that the serendipity of The Love Touch life within your excitement of your new-found life. Happy is Love Touching!

Let's move those personal wounds out of their social comfort zones and then not let them damage the psyche as much as the original wounds did. When we interrupt this destructive process with The Love Touch, we can move mountains. Wounds come from diversionary canals that drain water and spirit out of the river of our life. Having power over these negative levels of Cortisol will prevent continual diseases, depression, stresses, angers and cancers. These optimistic patterns that come from the Love Touch will change America. Let's start healing with constructive Love Touch today!

The Love Touch, Now!

The Love touch is necessary, because many of you have experience stresses that will drive a person to do hurtful things to them. Life hurts, and we do not know how to empty the body of stresses and traumas. We have a large amount of every day hurts with anger and depression that wound life! So on a day by day basis, we live in that loneliness Box and play the same nasty phases/broken records from our traumatic past. Stop it! Allow your mind to accept the goodness of daily touch and know that it can work for YOU!

MEC +1 Walk-in Clinic has great experiences: Tony from Chicago came to MEC+1 Clinic a number of times. When I looked into his eyes, he was handsome, because they had compassionate and caring. When I examined him, I noticed 2—3 degree burns on the right side of his face. I did not ask him, but he told me his wife in a gas explosion. He was sound with nerves of steel. He sat in the waiting room quietly. He was undoubted with how people viewed him. The MEC+1 clinic staff workers all want to talk to him when he came, because of his steadiness and caring attitude. He is not in the prison of hurt, fear, pain, sorrow, and anger!

I met Ceanuk, at a Washington D. C. charity dinner. Ceanuk was son historical family with an eight hundred chronicle and focused on saving his country! His needs were unselfish of pull the country together. I met him and he was kind, caring, very manly, but very compassionate! So, he was not imprisoned with self-talk pain!

Who is stressed, angry, lonesomeness, depression, illness? Stress has broken-records in their head. Record that play repeatedly! These poor life-style people need daily touch to free their wounded body and soul.

Many who are hurting, stressed, cool, lonely, angry, depression and ill? I need daily touch! You too can be steady and delightful and caring if you got touched and become healed.

You have been here, and how you know more than the average person in American. Why not share the love touch needs to be other! Blessings!

References

1. Field T: Touch. MIT Press, Cambridge, Mass., 2003.

2. Triplett J, Arneson S: The use of verbal and tactile comfort to alleviate distress in young hospitalized children.

    PERLINK "http://www.ncbi.nlm.nih.gov/entrez/ query. fcgi?cmd=Retrieve&db=pubmed&dopt= Abstract&list_ uids=254278"Res Nurs Health 1979; 126:101-110.

3. Schiffman HR: Sensation and Perception: An Integrated Approach. Wiley, New York, 1990.

4. Field T: Preschoolers in America are touched less and are more aggressive than preschoolers in France. Early Child Dev Care 1999; 151:11-17.

5. Schanberg S: The genetic basis for touch effects. In: Field T (ed): Touch in Early Development. Erlbaum, Mahwah, 1995, pp 67-79.

6. Schanberg S, Field T: Sensory deprivation stress and supplemental stimulation in the rat pup and preterm human neonate. Child Dev 1987; 58:1431-1447.

7. Escalona A, Field TM, Singer-Strunck R, Cullen C, Hartshorn K: Improvements in the behavior of children with autism following massage therapy. J Autism Dev Disord 2001; 31:513-516.

Field TM, Ironson G, Pickens J, Nawrocki T, Fox N, Scafadi F, Burman I, Schanberg S, Kuhn C: Massage therapy reduces anxiety and enhances EEG patterns of alertness and math computations. Int J Neurosci 1996; 86:197-205.

9.   Field TM, Hernandez-Reif M, Quintino O, Schanberg S, Kuhn C: Elder retired volunteers benefit from giving massage therapy to infants. J Appl Gerontol 1998; 17:229-239.

10.   Joan Borysenko-Massage Journal Interview, Fall 1999

11.   Rosa L, Rosa E, Sarner L, Barrett S. A Close Look at Therapeutic Touch. JAMA 279:1005-1010, 1998. To obtain a reprint of this article, send a self-addressed stamped envelope to the National Therapeutic Touch Study Group, 711 W. 9th St., Loveland, CO 80537.

12.   Nurse Healers-Professional Associates International. The Official Organization of Therapeutic Touch. The Nurse Healers-Professional About Therapeutic Touch page. Available at: http://www.therapeutic-touch.org/content/ ttouch.asp. Accessed November 22, 2002.

13.   Peters RM. The effectiveness of therapeutic touch: a meta—analytic review. Nurs Sci Q. 1999; 12:52-61.

14.   Gagne D, Toye RC. The effects of therapeutic touch and relaxation therapy in reducing anxiety. Arch Psych Nurs. 1994; 8:184-189.

15.   Keller E, Bzdek VM. Effects of therapeutic touch on tension headache pain. Nurs. Res. 1986; 35:101-106.

16.   Meehan TC. Therapeutic Touch and postoperative pain: A Rogerian research study. Nurs Sci Q. 1993; 6:69-78.

17.   Wirth DP. Complementary healing intervention and dermal wound reepithelialization: an overview. Int J Psychosom. 1995; 42:48-53.

18.   Turner JG, Clark AJ, Gauthier DK, et al. The effect of therapeutic touch on pain and anxiety in burn patients. J Adv Nurs. 1998; 28:10-20.

19.   Gordon A, Merenstein JH, D'Amico F, et al. The effects of therapeutic touch on patients with osteoarthritis of the knee. J FAM Pract. 1998; 47:271-277.

20.   Ireland M. Therapeutic touch with HIV-infected children: a pilot study. J Assoc Nurs AIDS Care. 1998; 9:68-77.

21.   Quinn JF. Therapeutic Touch as energy exchange: replication and extension. Nurs Sci Q. 1989; 2:79-87.

22.   Rosa L, Rosa E, Sarner L, et al. A close look at therapeutic touch. JAMA. 1998; 279:1005-1010.

23.   Pohl G, Seemann H, Zojer N et al. Laying on of hands" improves well-being in patients with advanced cancer. Support Care Cancer. 2006 Oct 13 [Epub ahead of print]

24.   Caroline Myss, myss.com, 1997

25.   1934-Wilhelm Reich-Austrian psychoanalysis. Freud's student. Used Somato techniques to dissolve muscular armor. Attempted to cure neuroses by releasing their corresponding muscle tensions by using breath, movement and physical manipulation. The community was outraged at the thought of using physical contact. He was sent to prison for his conflicts and died there.

Bioenergetics created by Alexander Lowen, emerged from Reich's work.

Also wrote "Joy-The surrender of the body to life", Depression and the Body: The Biological Basis of Faith and Reality "Depression has become so common that one psychiatrist even describes it as a "perfectly normal" reaction, provided, of course, it does not "interfere . . . ,

The "Language of the Body".

26.   Inkeles G. The New Massage. Unwin Hyman Ltd. Australia, 1981. Tarnould-Taylor W. Principles and Practice of Physical Therapy 4th ed. Stanley

27.   Thornes Ltd. UK. 1997.

      [Reference]. Encyclopedia Britannica. Oxford Unvisity Press, UK. 1996.
      [Reference]. Encarta. Microsoft, USA. 1997

      Lacroix N. The Art of Erotic Massage. Virgin, UK. 1994.
      Ylinen J., Cash M. Sports Massage. Stanley Paul, UK. 1988.
      Harris J. Swedish Massage: a Systematic and Practical Approach. Fowler, UK. 1983

28.   Egyptian Pictograph: ca. 2500 BC Integrity Bodyworks. 129 E Street-orange court, Davis CA 95616

29.   Scioli, A. (2006). Hope and Spirituality in the Age of Anxiety. In R. Estes (Ed.), Advancing Quality of Life in a Turbulent World. New York: Springer.

30.   http://www.holisticonline.com/ayurveda/ ayv—introduction.htm

31. http://massage-wire.com/news/news/the-massage:-a-brief—history.html

32. http://www.massagetherapylondon.com/index.php?p=28&pp=0

33. http://www.acupressureschool.com/massage_history.html

34. http://www.holisticonline.com/massage/mas_history.htm

35. http://massagetherapy.suite101.com/article.cfm/Historyofmassage

36. Oxytocin. From Wikipedia, the free encyclopedia.

37. Monday, 5 June, 2000, 13:33 GMT 14:33 UK. Japan 'the most healthy country' BBC

38. Stress Management Cortisol and Stress: How to Stay Healthy From Elizabeth Scott, M.S. Your Guide to Stress Management

39. About.com Health's Disease and Condition content is reviewed by Steven Gans, M.D.
     Cortisol and Your Body
     Diabetes in the US: a social epidemic
     By Peter Daniels
     30 January 2006

40. A cutaway view of human skin. The skin has two principle layers: the epidermis (a thin, outer layer) and the dermis (a thicker, inner layer). (Illustration by Hans & Cassady

41. Online Etymology Dictionary, massage

42. Merriam Webster Dictionary Online, massage

43.   Calvert, R. (2002-04-01). The History of Massage: An Illustrated Survey from Around the World. Healing Arts Press.

44.   Definition of massage, MedicineNet.com

45.   Massage Therapy as CAM. The National Center for Complementary and Alternative Medicine (NCCAM) (2006-9-01). Retrieved on 2007-09-26.

46.   Policy for Therapeutic Massage in an Academic Health Center: A Model for Standard Policy Development. The Journal of Alternative and Complementary Medicine (2007). Retrieved on 2007-09-26. 13 (4) pp.471-475

47.   A Meta-Analysis of Massage Therapy Research. Psychological Bulletin (2004). Retrieved on 2008-01-12.

48.   Massage Therapy. Harvard Men's Health Watch (2006-09-01). Retrieved on 2007-09-26. 11 (2) pp.6-7

49.   Massage Facts. National Certification Board for Therapeutic Massage & Bodywork. Retrieved on 2007-09-27.

50.   Potts, Malcolm, & Campbell, Martha. (2002). History of contraception. Gynecology and Obstetrics, vol. 6, ch. 8.

51.   C lcá in the Dic ionarul etimologic român, Alexandru Cior nescu, Universidad de la Laguna, Tenerife, 1958-1966

       MacGregor, H. (2004-12-28). Hospitals Getting a Grip: Massage Therapy Finds Place in Patient Care for FM and More. Los Angeles Times. Retrieved on 2007-08-31.

53.   Goodman, T. (2000-12-28). Massage craze: Hands-on therapy attracting more patients. CNN. Retrieved on 2007-08-31.

54.   Arnica Oil. Vitality Works. Retrieved on 2006-08-11.

55.   Automotive Engineering International Magazine Names Lexus LS 460 As 2007 Best Engineered Vehicle. SAE International (2007-04-10). Retrieved on 2007-05-06.

56.   Bowen Therapists Federation of Australia

57.   Lim SH, Anantharaman V, Teo WS, Goh PP, Tan AT. Comparison of treatment of supraventricular tachycardia by

       Valsalva maneuver and carotid sinus massage. Ann Emerg Med.
       1998 Jan; 31(1):30-5. PMID 9437338

58.   Ballo P, Bernabo D, Faraguti SA. Heart rate is a predictor of success in the treatment of adults with symptomatic paroxysmal supraventricular tachycardia. Eur Heart J. 2004 Aug; 25(15):1310-7. PMID 15288158

       Robertshawe P. (June 2007). "Massage for Osteoarthritis of the Knee". Journal of the Australian Traditional-Medicine Society 13 (2): 87.

60.   Calver, R. Pages from history: Swedish massage. Massage Magazine. Retrieved on 2006-12-25.

61.   Chia, Mantak & Maneewan. Chi Nei Tsang: Internal Organ Chi Massage. : Healing Tao Books, 1991. ISBN 0935621350.

62.   Evans, R. (2006). What Does the Research Say? Regents of the University of Minnesota. Retrieved on 2007-12-06.

       Muscolino, J. (2004). Anatomy of A Research Article. Massage Therapy Foundation. Retrieved on 2007-12-06.

64. Massage therapy for symptom control: outcome study at a major cancer center. NCBI PubMed (2004-09-12). Retrieved on 2007-09-11

65. Grealish L, Lomasney A, Whiteman B. (2000). Foot massage. A nursing intervention to modify the distressing symptoms of pain and nausea in patients hospitalized with cancer (abstract). PubMed NCBI. Retrieved on 2006-03-07.

66. Furlan A, Brosseau L, Imamura M, Irvin E. "Massage for low back pain.". Cochrane Database Syst Rev: CD001929. PMID 12076429.

67. Kuriyama, H. (2005). "Immunological and Psychological Benefits of Aromatherapy Massage (abstract)". Evidence-based Complementary and Alternative Medicine 2 (2): 179-184.

68. Massage for low back pain. NCBI PubMed (2002). Retrieved on 2007-09-28.

   Macgregor R, Campbell R, Gladden MH, Tennant N, Young D (2007). "Effects of massage on the mechanical behaviour of muscles in adolescents with spastic diplegia: a pilot study". Developmental medicine and child neurology 49 (3): 187-191. PMID 17355474.

70. Saltmarsh, S. (2006). "Voodoo or valid? Alternative therapies benefit those living with HIV". Positively Aware 3 (16): 46. PMID 16479668.

71. Kahn, J. (2005-06-10). Overview of Manual Therapy Use in the U.S. The National Center for Complementary and Alternative Medicine (NCCAM). Retrieved on 2007-09-26.

72. Stellin, S. (2007-07-15). Beyond the Body Wrap: What Makes a Spa Stand Out? New York Times. Retrieved on 2007-09-20.

73. States that require NCBTMB exams. National Certification Board for Therapeutic Massage and Bodywork. Retrieved on 2007-09-27.

74. What you n eed to know. National Certification Board for Therapeutic Massage and Bodywork. Retrieved on 2007-09-27.

75. Massage Therapy Law and Licensure and States Regulating Massage. Natural Healers. Retrieved on 2007-09-27.

76. Walsh, K. Massage craze: Hands-on therapy attracting more patients. Massage Magazine. Retrieved on 2007-08-31.

77. Verhoef, M. (2005-06-10). Overview of Manual Therapy in Canada. The National Center for Complementary and Alternative Medicine (NCCAM). Retrieved on 2007-09-26.

78. Sanders et al. (2003). "Use of Complementary and Alternative Medical Therapies Among Children with Special Health Care Needs in Southern Arizona". Pediatrics 111 (3): 584-587.

79. First-of-its-Kind Center Treats the Whole Person. Massage Magazine (2007-01). Retrieved on 2007-09-27.

80. Ellin, A. (2005-07-21). Now Let Us All Contemplate Our Own Financial Navels. New York Times. Retrieved on 2007-

Frank L. Clark, M.D.

I N K" h t t p: / / e n. w i k i P E d i a. o r g / w i k i /
September_20"\o "September20" 09-20.

81.   Crocker, Harry (2001-11-13). Triumph: A 2,000 Year
      History of the Catholic Church. Prima Lifestyles. ISBN
      07615292